THE

THRIVING

YOGA TEACHER

How To Create A Sustainable Career

Doing What You Love

MICHELLE LINANE

Creator of

Love Teaching Yoga

www.loveteachingyoga.com

DISCLAIMER

This publication contains materials designed to assist readers with personal advice in building sustainable careers for educational purposes only. While the author has made every attempt to verify that the information in this book is correct and up to date, the author assumes no responsibility for any error, inaccuracy or omission.

The advice, examples and strategies contained herein are not suitable for every situation. The materials contained herein are not intended to represent or guarantee you will achieve your desired results, and the author makes no such guarantee. The author shall not be liable for damages arising therefrom. Success is determined by a number of factors beyond the control of the author including but not limited to market conditions, the capital at hand, effort levels, and time. You understand every business idea carries an inherent risk of capital loss and failure.

This book is not intended for use as a source of legal or financial advice. Evaluating and launching a business involves complex legal and financial issues. You should always retain competent legal and financial professionals to provide guidance in evaluating and pursuing a specific business idea.

DEDICATION

To my soon-to-be husband, Ian. Your never-ending support of my dreams has been my anchor and is appreciated from the depths of my heart.

A special thank you to each of the teachers who opened their hearts and shared their stories with me. This book would not be the same without your love and wisdom. Thank you: Jen Wende, Courtney Mitchell, Charanpal Kaur, Yely Staley, Sarah Plummer Taylor, Allie Lehnhardt, Goldie Graham and Anna Guest-Jelley.

And to all the yoga teachers out there spreading the light. Your courage inspires me and your love has captured my heart. May you live an extraordinary life and leave your imprint on generations to come.

Namaste.

CONTENTS

FOREWORD

Teaching yoga invites us to delve more deeply into the practice of self-understanding in ways that enable us to share yoga with others in meaningful ways. The truly great yoga teacher keeps diving in, learning through his or her own practice along with deeper study of all of the foundational elements, from philosophy to the anatomy to seemingly mundane topics like sequencing and time management.

With years of experience one increasingly comes to appreciate that teaching yoga not only gives us this invitation but demands a lot of us, including with things that can seem anathema to yoga itself. If one wishes to truly thrive as a yoga teacher in the 21st century, it is rarely enough to only be a great teacher – one who fully shows up with clear intention, consistent motivation, an open mind and heart, and growing knowledge and skills. Along with these qualities, we need tools for successfully navigating the increasingly complex marketplace of yoga without losing our core values and heart-felt inspiration to teach.

When I first met Michelle Linane she was running Be The Change Yoga & Wellness, a successful studio she founded in northern California. There she created a space and a culture that allowed each and every teacher to be fully empowered not just in teaching, but in more fully living yoga- including in the ways that teachers learned how to best present themselves to their students and to the world. When Michelle was in my teacher training she immediately stood out as the one with keen insights into how we can best align our dreams with practical tools for making them come true. When we later worked together on a yoga business project, Michelle displayed not only great intelligence but the kind of creative thinking that is reflected in this wonderful gift of a book.

In these pages you will find the most well thought out ideas to translate your passion for teaching yoga into a successful profession sharing the practice of yoga in whatever ways you most imagine. She has not only more than done her homework, she has created a comprehensive and integrated manual for building a sustainable career as a yoga teacher. She shows you where to best place your time and energy, how to think big without losing your grounding, how to define and create balance in your business, and how to most fully, efficiently and effectively manifest yourself as a thriving yoga teacher.

If you are dreaming of having more of your life in the yoga world, if you are yoga teacher who wishes to make yoga the source of your livelihood, you have found your way to one of the best resources available. Enjoy it, savor it, put it into practice.

Mark Stephens
Author of *Teaching Yoga:*
Essential Foundations & Techniques

INTRODUCTION

Meet Jen Wende, world traveler, wife, mother and yoga teacher (www.jenwende.com). She's an inspiring example of someone who embodies the path of a teacher and is rocking her career. It must be said though, that it wasn't an easy road. Like so many of us, Jen stumbled upon yoga as a "broken person" years ago. In the emotional whirlwind of depression, a friend invited her to a yoga class at a local gym, and her life changed forever. During Savasana, the teacher read a quote so moving, Jen felt like the words were meant just for her. Walking out of the gym that day, Jen felt more relaxed and at ease then she could ever remember.

She was instantly hooked on yoga.

A few years later, no longer depressed, but still feeling discontent with her life, Jen embarked on journey to discover herself and the far reaches of the globe. Her travels brought her all over the world, including yoga teacher training in India and meditation study in Nepal. After 3 years, her travels abroad ended abruptly with a hospitalizing illness.

Upon returning home to Canada, Jen was on a wellness mission to regain her health and empower others to do the same.

After completing a coaching certification and yet another yoga teacher training, she took her first steps into the yoga profession. Starting small, she taught yoga to friends and family at home. Shortly after, she picked up some community classes at studios around town, but still kept a side job. One day, while working a catering shift, she met a Pilates instructor who became the catalyst to her next big steps as a full-time teacher.

As Jen puts it, she "dive-bombed into the deep end" of teaching full-time with group classes and private clients, subbing all over the city and "drowning herself in as many classes as she could teach". This was great for her learning experience and exposure to various teaching environments, but she didn't understand her value as a teacher. Saying yes to everything, and teaching from as early as 6:15am to as late as 9pm, was draining and made her unhappy. Oddly enough, at the time, she couldn't understand why she was so burnt out. Jen was comparing herself to a regular 40 hour a week job. So in her mind, 25 classes a week equated to 25 hours of work, which seemed like much less work than 40 hours. Unknowingly, Jen was misguiding herself by not taking into consideration the additional time and energy she spent in traveling to and from classes, the prep work involved, and the time spent before and after classes.

Slowly, Jen started waking up to the realization that her current path wasn't working. One day, as she weighed her empty bank account against her packed schedule, she couldn't understand why she wasn't making enough money to stay afloat. Her unhappiness didn't make sense and her eyes filled with tears. After all, she became a teacher for the balance yoga brought her, for the joy of sharing yoga with others, and freedom from the 9 to 5 job. How did she end up here?

Jen soon realized she'd had enough, but instead of walking away from teaching, she brainstormed options. Reflecting on her experience thus far, it came to mind that her students had been asking for additional offerings, such as guided mediations. Although she didn't know where it would lead her, Jen saw this as a way to diversify what she offered and the way she taught. She also considered the quality of her teaching. She wanted to help students more individually, so she focused extra effort on teaching private sessions.

However, it didn't take long before the reality of private teaching settled in. Yes, the compensation was better than group classes, but she was still running all over town and straining her energy. Jen then realized, she only had so many hours in a day, and with students wanting morning, lunch time and evening sessions, she couldn't fit in enough classes. Moreover, she still didn't have the freedom in her schedule she desired, so Jen explored her options yet again.

Contemplating her strengths and skills, she began to draw upon her previous career as an actress. It just so happened, Jen was leaving town for a few weeks and she didn't want to leave her clients hanging. Because of her experience acting, she felt comfortable in front of the camera and decided to film a video class for her clients while she was away. The response was great, and more opportunities arose. Although she wasn't charging yet for her videos, the idea that this could be her new path began to click. Soon after, Jen set out on a new venture to bring her teaching career online and expand her reach beyond her local community.

Of course this road had its ups and downs as well, but I'm saving the logistics of how she made this transition for later in the book. For now, I want you to reflect on Jen's story and how it relates to you. Where do you see yourself in her story? Has the challenge of earning a stable income teaching yoga ever brought you to tears? Does it ever hurt that the very thing you love so much can be so wearing on your soul?

I'm here to tell you that it doesn't have to be this way. You can have the yoga career you always dreamed of: fulfilling, purposeful and viable. If you're willing to think outside the box like Jen, I can help you create a career and life that you love. Just keep reading.

CHAPTER 1:
THE YOGA PROFESSION

Creating your dream career starts with understanding the profession. Jen's struggle is very common among yoga teachers, and sadly many will be dogged-down by the hardships. One factor in the equation is that teaching yoga isn't every teacher's true calling. Just like some of your fellow trainees in teacher training, some will explore the path, but veer in another direction. A larger part of the equation, however, is that teaching yoga isn't all peace, love and leggings. It's hard work. To truly make a living as a yoga teacher, you've got to think beyond the studio hustle. If you haven't witnessed this already, it's very rare that a teacher can survive on public classes alone. Think of a favorite local instructor who's well-known in your community. He or she likely facilitates their own teacher training, hosts workshops and retreats, and/or owns a studio. Now think about acclaimed teachers such as Seane Corn, Rusty Wells, Sadie Nardini, Kathryn Budig, and Mark Stephens. These teachers own studios, facilitate teacher trainings, and host workshops as well, but they've also written books, produced

DVDs, sell online courses, and speak internationally, among many other things. So, what's my point? Simply this: broaden your teaching horizons and you'll be well on your way to a sustainable career.

Now, I know what you may be thinking: Michelle, how am I ever going to be like Sadie Nardini? I know, I know, that's one lofty goal. But, I'm not saying *be* Sadie. Instead *think* like Sadie and start getting creative in the ways that you deliver yoga. The remarkable thing about being a yoga teacher today is you don't have to be a veteran celebrity teacher in order to make a living doing what you love. Thanks to the internet, you can build a tribe around the globe (or locally, for that matter) without having graced a single Yoga Journal cover. As Sadie puts it herself, "You have to believe you have a valid place in the yoga community. You are just as important as Patanjali" (Hurtado, J., Elephant Journal). I couldn't agree with her more. Each and every teacher has a role to play and a tribe to serve.

This book will show you how to branch out, attract your tribe and create multiple income streams for yourself. But, before we get into those actionable steps, there are a few more fundamentals about the profession to understand.

IS THIS YOUR SIDE JOB OR MAIN JOB?

The way I see it, we can categorize yoga teachers into two categories: those who need or want to make money teaching yoga and those who don't. The first type of teacher is anyone who depends on the income they make teaching yoga to pay the bills. They are the ones who teach full-time to earn a living or teach part-time as supplemental income to another job. Either way, they rely on teaching for income. The second category of teacher is anyone who has another job that provides their primary source of income or other circumstances put them in a position where they don't need to make money from the classes they teach.

It's important to be aware of which category you fall into, because this intention will show up as a driving force behind your financial decisions as a yoga teacher and understanding your value. As you may have observed, many yoga teachers have a hard time charging what they deserve to be paid. This pattern is common for many reasons, but we'll get to that in just a moment. Simply put, if you don't need to earn money teaching yoga to support yourself, then by all means, hook up your friends, volunteer, and don't shy from hefty discounts. However, if you're on the opposite end, this book will teach you how important it is to understand your value and intention behind compensation.

After contemplating where you fit in, there's a really important follow up question to ask yourself, especially if you depend upon the money you earn teaching yoga. Is teaching yoga something you want to turn into a career path? Although you are passionate about yoga beyond words, can you handle it becoming work? Many teachers struggle with this and rightfully so. For some, when their passion becomes work, over time it drains their love for it. However, for others like me, we just can't imagine a sweeter job than doing what we love for a living. So, think about it. Even if you don't depend upon the money to support yourself, teaching yoga can still feel like a job.

COMMERCIALIZING YOGA

Before we can get into the ethics of commercializing yoga, we must first understand what the word commercialization means. The commercialization of something is the process of introducing a service or product into commerce, which is the activity of buying and selling goods or services. Otherwise said, commercialization is bringing a good or service to market and often from small niche markets to mass markets.

Let's look at this term as it relates to food production in America. The commercialization of food production was a means to keep up with a rapidly growing population and demand after World War II. Fair enough, right? Would you be opposed to bringing food to everyone? Of course not. The problem of commercialization in food production lies within greed and exploitation. The intention of those in control was not purely to provide food to the masses. Oh no, they intended to make a huge profit and monopolize markets by taking food production out of the hands of small farmers and into the greased hands of a few large-scale productions. We now have a food system that caters to those at the top of the pyramid who care more about quantity not quality.

So what does this have to do with yoga? We could look at the commercialization of yoga in a similar light to that of food production. Don't we want yoga to be available to everyone, like food? Sure we do! We know the strength and wisdom in yoga and just about every teacher has stepped onto this path because they want to share the transformation of yoga with others. Not bringing yoga to the masses is like keeping it for ourselves or a select few markets. Like food production though, the challenge in commercializing something is that someone always wants to take advantage of an opportunity to make large commercial gains. In the process of making yoga more readily available, individuals, companies and organizations have begun to exploit it.

Unfortunately, this is almost always the case with bringing anything to the masses and can be considered a byproduct of the system. But what are we supposed to do as honest and gracious teachers? Forget about spreading the love and light of yoga because some will take advantage of its growing popularity? Are we supposed to stop eating food because of commercialized food production? No, that's absurd. But we can fight for changes in the system and make informed decisions about where and how we spend our dollars. The same goes for yoga.

Just because you're a yoga professional, doesn't mean you have to take part in the exploitation. You don't have to sacrifice quality for quantity as you share the practice and expand your reach. Yoga can be shared with the masses without the need for large-scale, corporate methods. Think of yourself like the small farmer bringing sustainable methods back into communities, cities and towns across America (and the world). Your intention isn't to greedily strip down yoga into a diluted and toxic form of what it once was in order to sell it to the masses, right? So, don't join those who are doing so and stay authentic to yourself and the teachings. We can't harbor the wisdom of yoga because we fear it will be exploited. That ship has set sail anyways. Instead, never stop exploring the practice and living the wisdom. Teach from your heart and what you know is right.

This world needs healing sooner rather than later. This world needs yoga and it needs you.

MAKING MONEY DOING WHAT YOU LOVE

Let me now address the taboo around money and yoga. As individuals with different upbringings and cultural backgrounds, we've all developed different relationships with money that may include debt, abundance, love, fear, lack, envy or desire. Layer that with the opposing views and attitudes towards money in the yoga world, and you'll see why it's no surprise many teachers struggle to pay their bills.

The thing about it is, we're experiencing a shift in modern yoga. Where the ancient practice was once a school of thought or tradition handed down through scriptures and spiritual teachings, the form of yoga today takes a much different shape. While it still remains true, that at the heart of what we are teaching is transformation from within, we live in societies that reflect a different way of life than the ancient teachers of the past.

History shows that human beings have engaged in trading since prehistoric times. What was once a method of bartering animals and grains to survive evolved into a system of trading coins, then paper money and now electronic debit and credit cards. What has remained throughout is the need for an effective tool to measure the value of goods and services being exchanged and whether you like it or not, the tool is money.

I want you to read the previous sentence again. The key term and a crucial ingredient in your recipe to make money doing what you love, is value. Value is a measure of the benefit that may be gained from a good or service. This is what so many yoga teachers forget, or don't know how to recognize- the value of the service we provide. There's no reason to feel guilt or shame for receiving money in exchange for the valuable service we perform. The exchange is fair. You give value and you receive value. Growing food and providing medical services are practices just as old as the ancient form of yoga, but these professions have adapted to the times as both farmers and doctors exchange their valuable services for currency in order to support themselves and their families. Comparing ourselves and monetary worth to teachers of the past, isn't serving us or our students well today. In our modern system of trade, we exchange currency for providing value, and we need that currency to put food in our mouths, clothes on our backs, and shelter over our heads.

Of course, that doesn't mean you can't do seva work too, but you have to make sure your basic needs are met. Don't forget, people are coming to you because they need your guidance and expertise, which you've invested a lot of effort, time and money into gaining. You deserve to earn a sustainable income and the more teachers are able to do so, the more people we can reach. Think of it like putting on your oxygen mask before assisting others. If you don't put your mask on first (i.e. earn a stable living to support yourself), you won't be as apt to help all those other people who need you, because you'll have to spend 40 hours a week at another job that pays the bills. You can't step fully into your power of teaching and serving, if you can't keep your own head out of water. As a reminder, I'll say it again, this world needs the healing of yoga, and we need you.

THINK LIKE AN ENTREPRENEUR

The entrepreneurial mindset is what keeps teachers in the game. Without making this shift in your thinking, you'll likely end up running in circles. I know from experience and in my heart that the more teachers learn to think with a business mind, the more people we are going to be able to help in this world. "This mind-set helps you maximize your time and talent to make a bigger impact on the world" (Demartini 71). That's all it is, a shift in your thinking to help you live up to your fullest potential. Don't let the word entrepreneur scare you. The way I'm about to break it down will actually inspire and empower you.

First, let's start with two literal definitions of an entrepreneur:

- A person who starts a business and is willing to risk loss in order to make money
- A person who organizes and manages any enterprise, especially a business, usually with considerable initiative and risk

Ok, maybe that does sound a little scary; business, risk, loss, enterprise! What? But fear not brave yogis, there's much more hidden in those definitions.

Look at the opening words in the first definition. An entrepreneur is a starter; an initiator or creator of a project, venture, or business. Someone who takes an idea and turns it into a reality. An entrepreneur is in the drivers' seat, and the one who propels the venture forward.

Let's look at some of the other words: organizes, manages and risk. An entrepreneur is also accountable and responsible for the destiny of their venture. They are willing to take risks and thus need to be fully empowered in order to direct the endeavor.

Now imagine your dream career as a yoga teacher. What does that look like for you? What does it feel like? What if you could turn that dream into a reality? Well guess what, you can!

By tapping into the entrepreneur mindset you can create the lush career teaching yoga you've envisioned for so long. You're already a leader by virtue of being a teacher, so embrace it and lead your career in the direction you dream of. No one is going to put together the pieces for you, so stop looking for external manifestation. You have to take initiative, create your own opportunities, and accept responsibility for your own career path. Standup for your dreams and be willing to take some risk in order to make them come true. It might feel unnerving, but you actually have the one thing that brings it all together. The special sauce. You have passion. Deep within, you have a burning desire to help others through the practice of yoga. It's your dharma.

Passion is what drives the entrepreneur and makes the risk worthwhile. Passion is the energy of your inner fire. It's the feeling you get when someone shares a heartfelt moment they experienced in your class. It's the force behind the transformation you've experienced from yoga, and the internal drive to help others find their transformation. It's what keeps you going despite all the challenges of the profession. Passion is the innate love deep inside the heart of an entrepreneur, so you my friend, already have the main ingredient. Now we just have to add to it.

THE MISSING INGREDIENTS

We can't talk about the entrepreneurial spirit without talking about business, and business skills are the missing ingredients to on-going success for many teachers. Passion without a plan, without action, and without hard work won't produce your dream career. **Lucky for you, passion isn't something you can learn, but business is.**

Consider this book the recipe to your ultimate teaching career. I'll help you blend your passion and profession with business savvy skills to pull it all together. You've likely got many of the necessary ingredients already in your cupboard. For some teachers it's just a matter of sorting through them, getting rid of what you don't need, and adding more of what you do need. For others, it'll be about learning new techniques and introducing new ingredients, and for some, we might be starting from scratch. Wherever you're at, it's important not to fear the word business either, as many teachers do. It's that fear-based mentality and misunderstanding of the term that is getting us into trouble.

Let's take a look at a few of the many definitions for the word business:

- An occupation, profession or trade
- A person, partnership, or corporation engaged in the trade of goods or services

- The practice of making one's living by engaging in commerce
- An affair or project
- Something with which a person is rightfully concerned

Why do yoga teachers fear business? If a business is just a trade, practice, or service, what in those definitions makes a teacher cringe and run for the hills? I think it's the words like corporation. Teachers often associate business with giant corporations, manipulative marketing, greed, and selling out. We see businesses exploit yoga for capital gain, and we don't want any part of it. The problem is, such businesses are motivated by increasing their bottom line instead of providing social benefit through the fruits of yoga.

However, the beautiful thing about business today is that businesses of all shapes and sizes are learning to value people over profit. Take Toms Shoes, for example. Doing good is the heart and soul of their business model, and making a profit comes as byproduct. These types of businesses are popping up across all markets from yoga to food to fashion.

You see, when your business actions and decisions are fueled by creating value for the people you serve, your business won't suffer from greed, deception or aggression. As yoga teachers, being of service is already what we do, so building a conscious business will come quite naturally once you release your fear of the ugly. Focus on the people you serve. Keep their best intentions in mind and let that be the driving force behind your actions. Do this, and you will no doubt attract abundance and a tribe of raving fans.

YOU ARE A BUSINESS

If you're sick of being underpaid and running around from studio to studio, then it's time to start thinking outside the studio. Ironically, one thing I learned from opening a studio is you don't need a studio to teach yoga. As part of my marketing efforts to draw people in, I was constantly out in the community giving people a taste of what we had to offer. I was also getting crafty with alternative ways to generate revenue for the studio. I got involved with farmers' markets, health fairs, fundraising walks, university clubs and events, community centers, non-profit organizations and corporate retreats. I created yoga programs for the city, small and large businesses, athletic teams, and even a local farm. Because all of those classes were taught on-site, I didn't need a physical studio and I quickly learned to think outside my own studio.

That being said, the studio itself served its own purpose and role in the community and I'm not devaluing that. Although, looking back on it now, I could have had an on-site yoga business without the overhead of a studio. When I was getting started, I didn't realize there were so many other ways of delivering yoga to the community, and I definitely didn't realize a teacher could be a business all on their own. In fact, according to the IRS, if you perform any non-employee work (teaching as an independent contractor or teaching private clients not contracted through a studio) you are self-employed and indeed conducting business on your own. Meaning, it's time to start thinking and acting like the businesses we are.

Breaking free from the studio hustle starts with viewing your profession as a legitimate business, and **thinking like a business gives you practical tools**

to maximize your potential and growth. Remember those definitions of business? You are an independent contractor trading yoga instruction and your career is your business. There's nothing wrong with thinking like a business savvy yogi. It's your career; it's your dharma that you're getting savvy about and you're in full control. Just because you're a business does not mean you have to step over to the dark side. Thinking like a business is simply a means of maximizing your potential to help you spread the light of yoga in a more effective and sustainable way.

There are unlimited opportunities to teach yoga, when you are willing to take the extra steps to create them yourself. The studio is not going to create them for you. Yes, it'll take more effort, organization and self-motivation. But, the benefits are far greater, and it doesn't mean you have to trade in your leggings for a pant suit. This book will walk you through the process of crafting your business savvy, heart-centered strategy to launch or elevate your own yoga business.

THINKING OUTSIDE THE STUDIO

Beside the fact it's hard to pay your bills teaching on a studio salary alone, there's a few more reasons to consider stepping outside the studio to build your career.

What will you do if the studio closes? Are there enough other options in your area to replace the income loss? What about all the other teachers who'll be displaced? Can the community absorb all of them into other facilities? Having been a studio owner myself, I can honestly say it's a very challenging thing to balance and make work in the long run.

How about the drop-in model most studios operate on? By the very nature of "dropping-in" to classes, students miss out on the benefits of committing to and planning time for a regular practice. Without committed students, the studio has to focus more energy on producing a regular flow of new students. I could go on further about how instruction, community, and impact also suffer on the drop-in model, but that's another story. What I want to point out is that drop-in studios usually generate inconsistent pay for teachers, which works against building a sustainable income for yourself.

What about competition and the constant turn-out of new teachers? Where do you think all these teachers will teach? Do you think our current system as a whole can handle the influx? What will happen when a new teacher is willing to work for less than you?

As I've mentioned, the studio hustle is no way to make a living. It's exhausting, leads to compassion fatigue and isn't sustainable in the long term. Let's look at some numbers to paint a clearer picture.

What's considered "full-time" as a yoga instructor varies greatly, but let's say you're a hustler and teaching 18 public classes a week. With most classes being at least 60 minutes in length, we can accommodate for the likelihood of at least a few of those 18 classes being 75 or 90 minute classes by giving this scenario a total of 22 hours of actual teaching time. Let's say you're also a teacher who shows up 15 minutes early to every class like I do. 15 minutes x 18 classes = 4 ½ more hours in a week. Now let's add in the 10 minutes or so it takes to wrap up and get out the door, 10 min x 18 classes = 3 hours. So, now we're looking at 22 + 4.5 + 3 = 29 ½ hours of your time dedicated to being at the studio or facility where you're teaching these public classes. Realize, I'm not even including the time it takes to drive back and forth and to plan/prepare your classes. Those two things could easily take another 5-10 hours a week. Remember how Jen was comparing her 25 classes a week to a 40-hour job, unable to understand her exhaustion? You can see how that comparison is extremely obscured, and she was likely working more than 40 hours considering all the variables with teaching yoga.

Ok, so we've got an average of 29 ½ hours a week of actual teaching time. Now, let's consider how much you get paid per class. The compensation rate of a yoga teacher varies significantly depending on where you live, so we'll break it down on multiple tiers. I'll take the amount you earn per class and multiple it by 18 classes to give us total weekly, monthly and yearly earnings. I'll then divide it by the actual number of hours worked (29 ½) to give you a true hourly rate. Here are some examples:

Rate Per Hour	Total Weekly Earnings	Total Monthly Earnings	Total Yearly Earnings	Hourly Rate
$15	$270	$1,080	$12,960	$9.15
$25	$450	$1,800	$21,600	$15.25
$35	$630	$2,520	$30,240	$21.36
$45	$810	$3,240	$38,880	$27.46
$55	$990	$3,960	$47,520	$33.56

(Figures shown reflect U.S.D.)

Sizing up the table above, keep in mind these figures represent 52 weeks a year, that's not deducting vacation time or taxes. If the top tier teacher paid 10% (which is a very conservative number) in taxes a year, they'd take home $42,768, not considering time off or paying for health insurance.

According to Career Trends, who gathers their data from government organizations, the average cost of living in the U.S. is as follows:

- Annual Cost for a Single Adult with No Children: $28,474
- Annual Cost for a Married Couple with One Child: $56,203
- Annual Cost for a Married Couple with Four Children: $82,900

Of course this is an average and many regions are much higher. You can check out the required income for your county using the Massachusetts Institute of Technology's Living Wage Calculator by visiting www.livingwage.mit.edu.

So, where do you fit in on the table above? Are you really willing to work for the hourly rate you fall into? Will your yearly earnings actually support you, and possibly a family? And even if you are one of the rare unicorns who make $55 or more a class, are you burnt out yet? Is 18 plus classes sustainable for your soul and basic needs?

Consider your current schedule. If you're a teacher currently leading less than 5 classes a week, but would love to take the plunge to teaching yoga full-time, does this outlook seem promising to you? Do you want your future to be teaching 18 plus classes a week (mornings, nights and weekends)?

If you're looking to increase your income as a yoga teacher, the answer isn't more studio classes. It's time to take initiative, branch out and create your own opportunities. Working smarter, not harder, becomes the name of the game. I'm talking about earning more per hour while freeing up your schedule (for those already teaching full-time) or filling up your desired schedule (for those looking to teach full-time). Private clients, workshops, corporate gigs, small private groups, online classes, public speaking, blogging and writing articles are all examples of thinking outside the studio. In the next chapter, we'll get into the details of diversifying, but first let's work through any fear you may be experiencing about creating your own yoga business.

CHAPTER 2:
DREAM BIG, LIVE BIG

"What would you attempt to do if you knew you couldn't fail" – unknown

The fear of failing keeps us playing small. Where your dreams might be quietly steering you to a stage as a motivational speaker, your fear screams that you aren't good enough and to stay where you are. But, what would you attempt to do if you knew you couldn't fail? Take the possibility of failure out of the equation and connect with what your heart truly desires. It's likely something bigger than you, so take yourself out of the equation too. Just like teaching yoga, it's not about us as teachers. It's about the students. How about this question: **what's truly worth doing whether you fail or succeed?**

Stories of success and achievement always begin with a big dream, and anyone who's basking in that glory will tell you there's nothing more important than casting aside your fears and reveling in your dream. As a yoga teacher, you're likely familiar with the power of visualization, so don't be afraid to imagine and daydream. People often shrug off their heart's desires as fantasy and the impossible. The reason why some people accomplish so little is because they never allow themselves to let go and just imagine the kind of life that is possible for them.

Meet Courtney Mitchell, elementary school teacher turned yoga teacher, the director of Experience Expositions and co-founder of The Yoga Expo (www.theyogaexpo.org). She's the kind of gal who bets on herself, dreams big, and lives big.

Upon completing her yoga teacher training, Courtney knew it would be her last year as a school teacher. In her transition to full-time yoga teacher, she started teaching yoga to her elementary students while saying "yes" to every other opportunity that came her way. Her original plan was to simply teach yoga full-time (anywhere and everywhere) because that's what her peers were doing. While that path served other teachers well, it didn't take long for Courtney to realize that course wasn't for her. As Courtney told me this story, she said, "You can't limit yourself to what those around you are doing". She wanted to do something different, something more. So, she opened her heart to possibility and the universe responded.

In another teacher training she met a gentleman by the name of Kyle who produced festivals. They began to work together brainstorming a yoga event for the community that would be different than all the other big yoga events out there. Their intention was something affordable, that could be brought to the masses, and focused on local teachers as opposed to celebrity teachers. With over 11,000 attendees at the first expo in their home state of Florida, classes were overflowing with participants and the vendor market was packed. It was a new experience for many teachers and they were elated by the opportunity of having an impact on such a big crowd. On a whim, they decided to book another expo in Los Angeles, California which has since lead to expos across the country. Talk about dreaming big! In just months, Courtney went from an average yoga teacher to the co-founder of a giant yoga event.

When I asked Courtney about the emotions she experienced during that transition, she humbly responded with, "The scary stuff is always the most rewarding. Say yes to whatever the universe gives you. If you really believe you can do it, you will do it. Even if it sounds crazy or people say it's unrealistic or you can't, it's only because they don't know how strong you are on the inside. You only fail when you stop trying". Be brave enough to live and learn, and don't let the fear of failure stop you from seeking your dreams. If it doesn't scare you (at least a little), it's likely your still playing small and staying in your comfort zone. As I always like to say, "Shoot for the moon, because even if you fall short, you'll still land among the stars". – Les Brown

OVERCOMING FEAR

"You can conquer any fear if you will only make up your mind to do so. For remember, fear doesn't exist anywhere except in the mind". - Dale Carnegie

Deep inside your heart, in those moments of a quiet mind, you know what you would love to be doing with your life and profession. You are here on this planet to achieve your greatest self in all areas of your life, and in order to realize your greatest self as a yoga teacher, you have to figure out what's blocking you.

One of the most common fears brought up in yoga teachers sounds like this: "Who am I to do this? Who am I to teach this knowledge? What do I have to offer?

If you find yourself stuck in this state of fear, I encourage you to ask instead, "Who am I NOT to do this?"

May I remind you, you are not the knowledge itself, but a channel through which the knowledge of yoga is shared. You have chosen the path of a teacher or maybe that path has chosen you. Commit yourself to the role and step fully into it with confidence, intention and love. You became a teacher because yoga changed you for the highest good. You have personally witnessed transformation within yourself and that is your credential and what inspires people. Who are you not to share that story and wisdom with people who need to hear it?

The Many Disguises of Fear

Our minds can be very sneaky, often working against what our hearts desire. When we dream and imagine the lives we long for, our minds often come up with a myriad of excuses that prevent us from taking action and fear takes over. I read the following on a music producer's blog once and the simplicity of his explanation has always stuck with me:

"Fear is a natural human response to unknown outcomes. As we take these situations into consideration, our minds make sure we have assessed the possible outcomes. This is human nature and a mostly positive survival instinct. However, there is a point where fear in our current context is given too much power. **That happens when we begin to fear the possible negative outcomes more than the potential gains**. Even worse, we begin to take on a dialog that hides these fears as something other than what they really are" (Blueprint).

Our fears become our excuses.

Our fears become our distractions.

Our fears become procrastination.

Our fears become our reality.

When we don't recognize a block as fear, it'll disguise itself as something else. Hidden deep down inside layers of emotions and self-talk, the fear of not being "good enough" often rises to the surface as one excuse after another, and we deny the fear itself. When you dream of writing a book one day, fear says: I'm not smart enough, I don't have the time, I don't have the money, or who in the world would even buy it anyways? When we sit down to outline our first workshop or event, fear says: I'm hungry, I have to check my email, people won't show up or I can't do it. When you think about creating a YouTube channel for your students, fear says: people won't like my voice, too many teachers are already doing it, no one will be interested in my videos, or I don't have what it takes to be in front of the camera.

Recognizing how fear shows up in you is the key to breaking through any block and actualizing the career you desire. When you're stuck in circles of excuses and distractions, you cannot see the truth in your heart. Like the gentle reminder of breath when we practice, continuously bring yourself back to your truth and "I can't" becomes "I can". As we gently bring our awareness back to the breath when the mind is distracted, we softly remind ourselves of our truth and the fear will start to fade with the excuses.

Henry Ford said it best, "Whether you think you can or you think you can't, you're right".

CHAPTER 3:
SHAPING YOUR BUSINESS

Let's recap the main points so far:

- Teaching yoga is hard work and it takes a lot of dedication to the practice, your students, and yourself
- If the income you need to keep a roof over your head comes from teaching yoga, you have to start thinking outside the studio
- Creating multiple streams of income is your key to financial freedom and a sustainable living teaching yoga
- Breaking free from the studio hustle starts with viewing your profession as a legitimate business, and thinking like a business gives you practical tools to manage your income streams and maximize your potential
- Understanding how fear may be blocking you from reaching your highest potential is essential to living out your purpose as a teacher

With that, we've laid the groundwork for understanding why a yoga business of your own is essential to a sustainable income as a yoga teacher. Now, we've got to figure out exactly what your business offers. Sure, you could simply offer yoga, but how many teachers, studios, community centers, and gyms already offer plain old yoga? They all do, so how will you be any different?

The key to standing out in a crowded space and building your business starts with connecting to your personal "why" and teaching intention. Why is it that you teach yoga? What brought you to the practice and inspired you teach? Getting clear on your intention for teaching yoga is fundamental to manifesting your dream yoga career. Think of it as your seed of intention. It is the starting point for which the growth of a tree begins, just as it will be the seed that creates the inspired career you dream of.

Writing Exercise

Grab your journal and something to write with. Find a quiet space and prepare for meditation. Sit in stillness for five minutes and let the mind quiet down. Feel free to light a candle, burn some incense, play some music, or anything that helps you tune-in and let go. Once you feel a state of deep relaxation, ask your heart what it deeply desires to share through the practice of yoga. Open your eyes and in your journal jot down everything that comes up: words, phrases, and even symbols or pictures if you please. Most importantly, don't think about it too much (remember, you asked your heart not your mind), let it flow honestly and don't fixate on any one response. When you feel like you've let it all out, put down the pen.

Now take a look at what you've written without judging yourself for any of it. Examine your words for similarities and what stands out to you. Look for clues of what originally guided you teach. Consider what most excites you about all the things you've written and what feels the most authentic to your heart desires? Connect with your "why".

YOUR TRADEMARK STORY

"Storytelling is the most powerful way to put ideas into the world today". — Robert McKee

Your trademark story combines your "why" and teaching intention. It plays an important role in not only crafting a niche for your business, but how you present yourself as a teacher. In essence, your trademark story becomes your credibility for teaching what you teach because it's your real-life experience. It's the reason behind why you do what you do. Your trademark story is your unique tale of transformation wrapped up into one easy to convey message.

Stories delight, touch, teach, recall, motivate and help us understand. Stories move us and make us feel alive. Your personal story is a powerful tool to connect emotionally with others. When people can relate to your story, they'll see themselves in it and feel empowered. Remember, you are your business, so it's vital that people know who you are and why they should put their trust in you.

Get in touch with what brought you to yoga and what eventually lead you to teach. What challenges or struggles did yoga help you overcome? How has it changed you? **The secret here is identifying a**

defining moment of transformation. Call it a moment of truth. A point in your story when the listener realizes the power in your message and feels moved to take action in their life too.

Your trademark story is part of your brand. Who you are and what you offer. It's distinctive to you and only you because no one else has the exact same life experience. It's your truth packaged in a way that only you can deliver.

In crafting your trademark story, here are the essential elements to include. Your story:

- Illustrates who you are
- Shows vulnerability
- Puts into words a defining moment of transformation
- Is relatable and draws people into the story
- Demonstrates the potential and value you can bring to the listener's life too
- Explains why a person should choose you

Your story of change and transformation can heal you and others, so express it. Sit down and journal it out. Go through the previous teaching intention exercise and let your heart speak through your pen.

Then share it with someone and practice conveying your message. This will help you refine it into a concise elevator pitch so to speak, while boosting your confidence in speaking your truth. It doesn't have to be glamorous or traumatic, it just has to be real and reflective of the human experience.

These defining moments of change usually influence how we teach and what we become passionate about in yoga. Open your heart and get in touch with what's inside. If it moves you, it'll move others. Through connection and transformation, your personal story paves the way to your successful yoga business, so don't take a shortcut.

CARVE OUT A NICHE

Now that you've connected with your personal "why", think about how that may shape your niche. For example, a friend and fellow teacher who had a stroke at the age of 29 used yoga to regain movement in the right side of her body. She now teaches yoga for stroke recovery patients at local hospitals and with private clients. Think about how you can use your passions, personal interests and life experiences to find your specialty and separate yourself from the pack.

Most new teachers take any teaching opportunity that comes their way in an attempt to gain as much experience as soon as possible. What they are essentially doing is promoting themselves as a jack-of-all-trades, and often fall short due to a lack of experience. While I do agree with exposing yourself to as much teaching experience as you can, it's crucial to specialize in something when building your yoga business. The idea is to create a brand or a position for yourself in the marketplace that people need and can remember. Yoga is a crowded industry, but a niche makes you the big fish in a small pond.

I know it sounds scary to narrow your audience down to one group, but it actually simplifies your business, I promise. **With a niche, you're not turning away students, you're attracting your tribe.** Yoga Journal, Yoga Works, and Prana seem to have something for everyone, but that's just not practical for the small business. You have to start by focusing on one group. Not to mention, having a group of people you really enjoy working with takes the pressure off of having to appeal to the masses- you don't have to be liked by everyone. A niche gives you the freedom to be authentic and stay true to the vibe that will attract your tribe.

When you niche down, you become known as an expert and the go-to person in your community. It brings clarity to your business strategy and liberates you from the confusion and guesswork of trying to appeal to everyone. When everyone is your preferred audience, your message gets watered down and the quality of your service and expertise diminishes. When you try to be everything to everyone, you end up talking to no one.

In working with a niche, your marketing and networking efforts become more efficient and effective. For instance, you'll know what workshops, trainings, and conferences to attend, as well as what businesses to partner with. You'll know exactly what to say when someone asks about your work and your outreach becomes a breeze because you know your audience so well.

Whether you have a niche already or you're figuring it out, it's essential to get extremely specific. As marketing expert Derek Halpern puts it, "You have to drill down to exactly what you want to be known for and sum it up in a few words".

When selecting a niche for your business, ask yourself the following questions:

- The students who give me the most positive feedback in my classes are_____.
- Of all the people who could use my service, who am I most passionate about working with? Who do I most identify with, understand and even sympathize with?
- What do I love to talk about more than anything?
- What about yoga most excites me?
- What specialized training do I have and how can I use that to shape my niche?
- I'm naturally really good at _____.
- My students love _____ about me.

Remember, you're carving out a role as an expert and the go-to teacher for something specific. Don't try to master two or three niches at once (i.e. senior yoga, yoga for athletes and kids yoga). The way you speak to and market yourself to seniors is going to be completely different than athletes or kids. Gain experience in one area first, learn from your wins and mistakes, and establish your authority. Then develop a second niche if that suits you or transition to something else if that's the way life is guiding you. Nonetheless, get really good at one thing initially, and then expand. Think about Nike, a company that produces just about every type of athletic shoe. They didn't begin that way, though. First, they carved out a niche for their brand by dominating the running shoe. Over the years Nike has added to their repertoire niche by niche to the multifaceted company they are today.

In crafting your niche, the formula is simple: **Need + Solution = Niche**. First, identify a need among a specific group or community. Then identify what their biggest pain/obstacle/challenge is, and come up with a way to help them resolve it.

Here are some niche examples:

- At home prenatal yoga for working moms-to-be
- Restorative yoga for CrossFit recovery
- Yoga and Ayurveda for digestive healing
- Bikram Yoga for athletes
- Team building yoga for corporate retreats
- Yoga for men with athletic injuries

- Yoga and creative arts for at-risk teen girls
- Yoga to balance depression
- Yoga for seniors with hip replacements
- Strengthening yoga for ballet dancers with joint instability
- Corporate yoga to improve posture and reduce stress

Choose a niche you are actually qualified to teach. That is, you have the technical knowledge to skillfully address the needs of your niche. The idea is to become an expert in your niche, not a fake. These days there are teacher trainings for almost every specialty, so acquire the related certifications, conduct your own research, learn as much about your specialty as you can and grow from your experience. Remember, the best teachers never stop exploring their craft, and that's what it takes to become a great teacher in any niche.

TEACH PEOPLE WHO DON'T PRACTICE YOGA

Studios are missing out on a big percentage of the population: those who haven't or don't practice yoga. For these folks, a large majority will never step foot in a studio because they're intimidated, aren't flexible already, or don't feel they fit the stereotype. Many are aware of the benefits, but because they still aren't sure if yoga is for them or they can't find specialized classes that fit their unique needs, will never attend a studio class regardless of the Gentle, Beginners, Slow Flow or Intro To Yoga title we give it.

This presents a unique situation for yoga teachers who are looking to teach outside the studio. There are so many ways to reach people who aren't already practicing yoga. The key is to understand how to reach them, and to meet them where they already are. Connect with your audience where they feel comfortable: on the golf course, at work, in their home, and by partnering with businesses who already serve them. I've touched upon this a bit already, but here lies an opportunity to really get out in the community. To serve people who aren't being served. All the while carving out a unique space in the community to build yourself a sustainable career.

ASK, DON'T ASSUME

Figuring out exactly what the pain points are of you niche market is a crucial step that many people skip. Simply identifying a group of people you want to work with isn't enough. You have to know how to help them *and* what they really need help with. You have to ask people what is happening in their life that presents a major challenge for them, and get to know their struggles by talking with them. Yep, that's right; I want you to have actual conversations with folks in the niche group you want to work with. Don't just assume you know what they need. Believe me; taking the time to complete this step in the beginning will save you a ton of time in the long run. Here's why it's important to ask:

1. If you don't know what the pain points are for your niche, asking people will supply you with accurate information.
2. If you think you already know the pain points of your niche group, asking them will either validate what you thought or steer you in the right direction.
3. Talking with actual people in your niche group will write your marketing copy for

you. You'll know how to present what you offer in their own words, which assures them that you truly know how to help them.

4. The folks you are talking with are also potential clients. In having these conversations, you begin to establish relationships that can turn into paying clients. Once you've developed a way to help them, you can return to these individuals and present your solution. It's likely they know other people facing the same challenges too, which can be helpful when you're looking for referrals to do your research asking, as well as finding paying clients once your business is ready.

Now, you're probably wandering how you find people in your niche to talk to. It could be a group of people that you're already connected to, so scheduling coffee shop chats will be easy. On the other hand, you might need to do some research to find them. Start with your network: people at work, your family, Facebook friends, the parents of your children's friends etc. Find out if any of these people are in your niche group, in addition to asking them if they know other people who are. For example, say you want to help golfers improve their game by opening up the hips and shoulders with yoga. Ask those in your immediate network if they golf and ask them to refer their golf buddies to you as well.

If you don't get enough contacts that way, use Facebook groups and blogs. In the golf illustration, look up golf groups on Facebook and read the group discussions. Find people who show concern for improving their game and reach out to them. Let them know you're conducting research and would love to chat with them briefly (in person, on the phone or via Skype) about what obstacles are in their way. You could also find popular golf blogs and read the comment sections on articles that discuss matters around improving one's golf game. If you find someone through a comment who could be a good fit, reply to their comment, explain your situation and ask if you can reach out via email.

Another way to find people in your niche is to locate other businesses that work within your niche. In the golf scenario, you could go to a golf course to seek out people to talk with. I've personally worked on a golf course before and can say the vast majority of the folks working there love golf, so talk to cart guys and other employees in the golf shop and restaurants.

If you are wandering what to ask people, I've found the POD technique from Derek Halpern, expert marketer and entrepreneur, works wonders. POD = Problem, Obstacle and Desire. In the words of Derek himself, here's how he explains the POD technique as heard on episode 184 of The Smart Passive Income Podcast with Pat Flynn (www.smartpassiveincome.com/podcasts/psychological-strategies-to-improve-email-conversion-with-derek-halpern):

PROBLEM

> *"Thing #1 is the problem that this person has in their life right now that they want solved. I always say you want to start with the problem because if people have a problem in their life right now they're going to want to cure that problem. If you don't start with the problem, you might fall for the trap where you create something that you think people should want, but they don't want yet because there's no pressing problem in their life to solve it.*

There was an article that I read recently about why start-ups fail, and it was something like 70% of these start-ups failed because they created a product that they thought people should want, but they had no reason to buy."

DESIRE

"Now, the third thing – I know I'm skipping #2, but we're going from 1 to 3. The third thing you want to find out, which is actually the 2nd thing you find out (but it doesn't spell a nice word when you go PDO) so, the third thing you want to find out is the desire that person has.

Again, start with the problem in their life. Now you want to talk to them and find out the desire they have, like this is the problem in their life, and what would their life look like in an ideal world? That's the desire. You want to talk about the end result that people have."

Let me give you an example. In the golf scenario, when you ask someone what their biggest pain point is with golf, you might hear something like, "I need to open up my swing". Ok, that's the factual problem they are currently facing. Now, what would their life look like in an ideal world? You can literally ask them that, and you may hear something like, "Well for starters, I'd stop losing to my brother all the time". Winning is the end result and beating his or her brother in the game is the desire.

Ok, let's get back to Derek:

> *"So you want to focus on the desire. The desire isn't to solve the problem; the desire is what happens if that problem doesn't exist? What does their life look like? How great is their life? How miserable is their life? Maybe it's more miserable, I don't know, but you want to start with the problem and the third thing you want to get is the desire that they have. Then, here's where the fun comes into play. Once you know the problem and you know the desire, now you need to catalog the obstacles*

standing between the problem and the desire."

OBSTACLE

"These could be all sorts of obstacles. There could be mindset stuff. There could be, "I'm scared to do this". That's one obstacle. Another obstacle might be, "I don't have the money to fix this problem". Another obstacle might be, "I don't have the time to fix this problem". You want to go through these lists of obstacles.

When you're talking to your ideal customers you want to find the problem, you want to find the desire, and you want to try to get an exhaustive list of all the different types of obstacles that your potential customers are going to encounter while they're trying to cure their problem and end up in their desire."

Using our golf example, one obstacle that might come up is, "I practice all the time, but my golf swing just doesn't improve. I don't think there's anything else I can do". Another one might be, "I can't afford to work with a personal golf coach" or "My brother is just better than me, I'll never beat him".

> *If you look at all the best sales people, best copywriters, and best people in the world that do this stuff, the one thing that they all have in common is that they know the customer better than they know themselves. You can't know the customer better than you know yourself unless you do this. You have to use the POD technique to understand who you're talking to.*

Here are a few more tips to help you along the way with the POD technique:

- **Don't be afraid to hear that your idea isn't really what people need.** Doing this part of the work helps you create something that will truly benefit someone else, as well as your business. It'll be far worse to find out your idea won't sell after investing a ton of time, energy and money into it.

- Build rapport with the people before diving into their pain points. Introduce yourself, share a moment of personal vulnerability, and make yourself relatable. Keep in mind their best interest and don't be manipulative. Try to inspire them by revealing a bit about yourself.
- Let them know this is personal research, and you won't be quoting them or publishing their story.
- Ask plenty of open-ended questions. Let people tell you the truth, and stay away from accidently steering them in the direction you want or confining them to only a couple of answers. PRO TIP: the people who have long answers and spend the most time with you are your target audience. They're the ones who'll be ready to sign up with you when you're ready to take on clients.
- Ask and have this discussion with at least 5-10 different people.

MARKET RESEARCH

What I just outlined with pain points and the POD technique is essentially doing your market research, but there's still more you can do. In conducting market research you'll gather information about current trends in your niche, competitor information, and you'll get to know your target audience even better. It's a process of understanding what is in demand and how competitive a niche is in effort to reduce risk, spot potential problems, and identify opportunities. What the POD technique gives you is called primary research: interviews and first-hand experiences. Secondary research is finding data that is already compiled for you: statistics, demographics, reports, government data, etc. Both are important and both can mean the difference between succeeding in the long run or not.

Use some of the same strategies for finding people in your niche that I suggested above. Join Facebook groups, follow blogs, and check out online forums that cater to your niche group. You can even search Amazon for books on your niche and read the reviews for evidence of what people are finding useful and are still looking for. Use these platforms to learn more about your group, how they communicate to one another, what's their average age range, what are their other interests, and what's their average income? A heart-wrenching question to explore is, are they a group who is willing to and can afford to pay for the service you want to offer? This is a huge issue to address. I've actually seen it play out as the downfall to a business. A friend created a business around a demographic who couldn't afford to pay for it. I know that brings up a lot of mixed feelings, but hey, if you're a teacher who needs to earn an income from your business, this is an essential matter to mull over.

HELPFUL WEBSTIES FOR MARKET RESEARCH:

1. U.S. Census Bureau (www.census.gov)
   Use this resource to access info about people, businesses, geography, trade and much more.
2. Quick Facts (www.quickfacts.census.gov)
   This easy to use website provides fast access to a wide range of info about population on the state, county or city level.
3. Statistics Canada (www.statcan.gc.ca)
   Provides data about Canada compiled by the Canadian government. Search a wide variety of subjects, demographics, reports and articles.

4. The World Bank (www.worldbank.org)
   This international organization compiles data worldwide. It offers free data by topic or country, contains links to online databases, and publishes its own economic reports.

I can't express to you enough how important it is to speak directly to people in your niche and conduct market research on your niche. **The trick to standing out in a crowd isn't flashy flyers or a shiny website.** Across all industries, what separates successful businesses from those who are barely getting by is this step. Find out what people really need and don't just assume.

BECOME AN EXPERT

Becoming an expert in your niche is about establishing yourself as a community or industry leader. This doesn't mean you have to know everything and stand as the be-all, end-all. You just have to be the one willing to do the research and pull information together from various resources into one convenient space. An expert is simply a person who has comprehensive and authoritative knowledge in a particular area. It's simply taking your role as a teacher in a niche community to a higher level by developing credibility in the space as a whole.

People trust experts, so developing your expertise will help you stand out as the best person to help them. Expert content marketer and SEO strategist, Eric Enge explains, "A deep understanding of your topic makes you more trustworthy, and that makes you the more inviting choice when it comes time to purchase a product or service. This is particularly true if you combine being an expert with a strong sense of ethics" (Copyblogger).

In developing your expertise, you'll acquire more knowledge and skills you can use to truly help people. Likewise, it'll help you understand your business better. When you really know your subject and niche, you can run your business more efficiently. For example, creating marketing content for your business will be a whole lot easier when you know the ins-and-outs of your niche.

A few more reasons to develop your expertise include:

- Experts call for higher pay
- Other experts or businesses in your niche will want to collaborate with you
- Communities will form around you
- Experts are often asked to join events, speaking engagements and panels

Start by reading the top selling books in your niche. In addition to absorbing the information in these books, seek out other resources from top performers in your niche. Subscribe to blogs and publications that relate to your niche and regularly read their content. Attend related conferences, seminars and events, and be sure to take any available teacher trainings or online courses.

As you deepen your understanding, the next step is to begin sharing your knowledge and message. By simply sharing your information, people will start to recognize you as someone who knows a lot about your topic. The more you share, the more people in your niche will recognize your name and your status will grow organically. There are numerous fun and creative ways to share your message and expertise. Here are a few to help you establish yourself:

- Start a blog and write original content pertaining to your niche
- Write and submit articles to top publications such as Elephant Journal and use your bio to link back to your website/blog
- Guest-post on blogs from other leaders in your niche
- Find local events in your area that relate to your niche and offer to speak on the subject or teach a class
- Reach out to other businesses that serve your niche to cross-promote and collaborate
- Speak at local college and university events, partner with campus clubs or the student health center, and ask individual professors if you can speak or guest teach in their class
- Teach a seminar or class at a related non-profit organization or other business
- Join forums and Facebook groups related to your niche and provide value by engaging in conversations and providing helpful information

To help you imagine this a bit more, let's revisit our golf scenario from the Ask, Don't Assume section. If you recall, in this example, your niche is helping golfers beat their buddies by improving the range of motion in their swing and their mental focus. Your first step is to create your own hub in the internet land where you showcase your expertise and services (aka, your website and blog). Use your blog as a way to drive traffic and provide helpful information to students, potential students, and general value to the niche as a whole. Another great online resource is podcasts. Get on iTunes and search for golf and yoga podcasts. Reach out to the host and propose an idea featuring you and your expertise for a show.

Next, write and submit articles to major golf publications, such as Golf Digest and Golf Magazine to boost your credibility and link back to your website, as well as yoga publications like Yoga International. With the need for so much online content these days, it's actually easier than you think to get your articles published. Similarly, reach out to golf and yoga blogs and offer to write content as a guest-post on their blog. As before, use the opportunity to drive traffic to your website by linking back to it, and to build your credibility and resume.

Now, for the in-person stuff. Google "golf events" in your area and explore how you could bring your expertise and yoga to these events. A search in my local area yielded a ton of results from tournaments to charity events to golf clinics. I also found local coaches, courses, shops and clubs that one could potentially partner with. I even found a mixer event at a nearby golf course, and if you aren't familiar with mixers, they are hosted specifically for networking and introducing people in a community to one another. Perfect! You could also seek out golf teams from high school to college to adult leagues.

PRO TIP: Know that all this effort establishing your expertise, is simultaneously serving your marketing plan. While you are speaking at a golf symposium or teaching a class prior to a tournament, you're promoting your service to everyone in attendance. This will no doubt, yield some business right off the bat. As you partner with a golf shop, ask to set out your business cards or write a short promo for their next newsletter. The opportunities are endless and often, you don't know what's even possible until you get out there and start talking to people. People in other areas of your niche will have ideas that never crossed your mind and will help you learn more about how you can serve this unique community even better.

Lastly, being an expert means that you never stop exploring your craft. Only a fool assumes they know everything there is to know about a particular topic. Being an expert means that you are someone who is constantly on the move and learning. Explore as much as you can, become a trusted resource and be helpful to others in your niche space.

CHAPTER 4:
MULTIPLE STREAMS OF INCOME

Ok, so now you're thinking like an entrepreneur and treating your career like the legit business it is. You've identified a niche and have talked with real people to find out exactly what their pain points are and how you can best help them. You've also started to build your credibility and make connections in your niche space. Now what?

I'll let you in on a little secret, the average millionaire has at least seven different streams of income. Compare that with the average American whose income relies primarily on one day-job, and it's no wonder why wealthy individuals build wealth faster than the average person. Now, I'm not implying that you should strive to be a millionaire, but in your efforts to build a sustainable income, there's a lot to be learned from the behaviors of millionaires.

The next step to building your badass yoga business is figuring out how to take what you have to offer and diversify it into multiple services and income streams. It's helpful to start by differentiating between types of income, so you can understand the two basic categories: active and passive income.

Active income is how people traditionally view income, as a salary or hourly wage, with the primary component being your time. It's income that is generated by a direct trade of your time for a specified wage. All the in-person classes you teach (whether private or public) require you to actively be there in order to earn the agreed upon income, and are forms of active income.

Passive income is much less traditional and is not a form of trading direct hours for dollars. Passive income is income received on a regular basis with little effort and time to maintain. An example you are likely familiar with is investing into stocks or bonds. You earn from dividends and interest, and there's little to no work done on your part aside from checking every so often to ensure your investments are performing the way you hoped. It's passive because you aren't directly trading your time for the money you earn.

Do I think yoga teachers should invest their money into stocks, retirement funds and rental properties? Yes, of course. Investing can be a huge part of anyone's income, but that's not for me to advise you on. This chapter will give you some ideas about how to create multiple streams of income that are both passive and active, but all related to teaching yoga.

Let's start with what we're most familiar with, active income.

ACTIVE INCOME

Public Classes

Yes, I want you to think beyond studio classes because it's not financially feasible to put all your time into them, but they are still a means of income worth talking about. Some studios actually pay really well and are monetarily worth keeping. There's also a few other reasons to consider keeping a few studio classes on your schedule:

- They are an excellent way to build your local following
- Being a familiar face at the studio will help you fill up workshops and events
- Attending students can convert into private clients with a little promotional effort from you
- Your regulars may refer their friends to you
- Your in-person students are a great place to start promoting your online classes or other services such as counseling or Reiki

If you're a teacher who has a schedule jam-packed with studio and gym classes, take a serious look at those classes and deicide which, if any, make sense to keep and humbly say goodbye to the others so you have time in your schedule for other streams of income.

PRO-TIP: An often overlooked way to increase your income immediately is to ask for a raise from your studio classes. People across all professions go years without receiving a raise, and not because they don't deserve it, simply because they didn't ask. Be professional about it, know your worth and then demonstrate that worth to the owners.

Private Clients

Teaching private yoga requires a different talent than group classes, and can shape you into a more skilled teacher. Instead of teaching from a generalized group sequence, you'll learn to teach from your student's needs, strengths and limitations; a skill that separates the greats from the mediocre. Teaching a personally tailored sequence also enables you to have a greater impact on your student's health and well-being. But that's not all folks, teaching private yoga allows you to earn more per hour than teaching studio classes. Depending on your area, niche and quality of service, you can charge between $75 and $200 per hour/session.

You can also take your pricing for private sessions in a different direction with what I like to call value packages. With value packages there's not only potential to earn more, but you also get the opportunity to integrate some of your other gifts like Reiki, massage therapy, or essential oils. The common method of packaging private sessions is to offer a discount incentive to purchase bundles of classes upfront. The difference in value packaging is that the packages differ not by the number of sessions, but by the value of what clients receive. With value packaging each pricing tier offers more value through additional services and support like a mediation download or counseling sessions. For more detailed information and examples of value packaging please see the Value Packaging section in Chapter 7.

Independent Group Classes/Series

Offering independent group classes is another way to earn more and build your local following. When I say independent group classes, what I'm referring to are classes that you host and build on your own, outside the studio. You could rent space by the hour at a local community center, event/banquet hall, church, wellness center or non-profit, to name a few options. Because your personal money is on the line with space rental and marketing, I don't recommend offering weekly drop-in classes because they're inconsistent and lack student commitment. Instead, with independent group classes offer a series for a specified period of time and the class fee is paid for upfront.

For example, if your niche is yoga for runners, you could offer a four-week series to build stronger knees and open the hamstrings. First, determine what your time is worth, how much you would need to earn to cover your costs and make a profit. Then figure out how many students that will require and what their individual cost would be. The beauty of a class series is that folks who can't afford the higher price tag of private sessions still receive individualized attention and specialized classes that aren't offered in studios.

Let's say you charged students $80 for a four-week series. If it were an hour class once a week that would be $20 per class for the student. Depending on where you live, that may be the same cost as a studio drop-in or only a few bucks more, and a whole lot cheaper than a private. If you got 6 people to register, your net revenue would be $480. If your space rental was $25 an hour, subtract $100 for the four weeks and you'd profit $380. That breaks down to $95 a class, which for the average teacher, is much better than your studio pays you per class.

There are many other benefits to small groups and class series. When you rent space from an established organization like a wellness center, there's a high probability they'll let you promote your classes to their community. That's a huge head start when you're just beginning to grow. You'll also be supporting the business or organization by renting the space, which is added revenue for them as well. Lastly, with a series, students pay upfront and commit to all the sessions which has multiple benefits in itself:

- You can theme the series and progress with confidence, as everyone in the class will have attended the previous class
- Because noticeable shifts and results often take time, you'll have a higher success rate because students are committed to the specified duration and not just dropping-in from time to time
- Since the same students will attend for the whole series, people get to know one another and support and motivate each other, which builds a stronger sense of community
- Because you aren't committing to a regular class, week in and week out, you build freedom into your schedule and can host a class series when it's convenient for you

Workshops & Events

Workshops and events are awesome ways to go deeper into themes and topics, as well as integrate your other skills and passions, such as dance or meditation. They're also great for supplemental income and can even be excellent sources of steady income if you like to travel and don't mind working weekends. To really optimize your business and marketing efforts, keep your workshop themes within your niche. Feel free to explore various venues to host your workshop or event. Once again, teachers often feel restricted to studios, but when you have a specific niche, it's easy to branch out and still fill your event. Let's say your niche is prenatal yoga, a few places you could host a workshop or event are: birthing centers, hospitals, private medical offices, wellness centers, chiropractic offices, moms groups/meetups, and other like businesses or organizations that work pregnant women.

Workshops are great because you'll earn a big chunk of cash all at once, but you have to play your cards right, save and budget accordingly. In creating your workshops, know if you want to offer a premium workshop or something more budget friendly, because the work you put into it and the resources you provide will vary. I find it's helpful to have both, so you can accommodate different studios and venues. Again, so much of workshop pricing depends on the location and your niche, but as you start to travel, do your research and choose wisely. A premium workshop upwards of $150 won't fly at any old studio. You have to find a studio that not only has regular students within your niche population, but also students who can afford it and will see the value in the price tag.

Another key element to boosting your income with workshops and events is scalability. That is, being able to handle the workload of growing your workshops and events with ease. Your workshop(s) should be repeatable and require less time to prepare each time you host it. By simply changing the location, date and time you can use the same marketing materials saving you tons of time. Rinsing and repeating the same workshop gives you time to work out the kinks and improve it to the highest quality you're capable of. Call it a signature workshop or event, it'll help you grow your niche following and reputation as the go-to person within that space.

Teach Corporate Gigs

Corporate yoga (sometimes called workplace yoga) is a booming market with the recent growth of employee wellness programs. Businesses are recognizing the value of prevention and caring for the well-being of their employees beyond medical (sick) care. This produces a huge opportunity for yoga teachers building their own business. With a website and some brochures, you can create your own corporate opportunities. If you're willing to do the legwork, it'll pay off handsomely.

Corporate and workplace classes call for a higher price point and are generally consistent gigs. Again, depending where you are, small businesses can bring in $65-$100 per class, while higher profile companies can bring in $110-$200 a class. Like private sessions, value packaging can come in handy with corporate yoga. You can build more value into your corporate classes by offering more than just yoga, such as massage therapy.

Specific programming can also be of benefit to help you land a corporate gig. Instead of plainly offering yoga, get more creative and detailed. Offer a program for reducing stress, improving posture, preventing back pain or injury, alleviating carpal tunnel syndrome, or counterbalancing repetitive movements. Do some investigation on the business you'd like to approach, try to find out what their employees need most, and propose a few ideas. In your programming, also include the duration and frequency of classes, and the program length (6 weeks, 3 months, 6 months etc.).

I think this goes without saying, but it's crucial to present yourself professionally. At the very least have a business card and resume. Moreover, brochures, a website and printouts outlining your programming will boost the company's confidence in you. Be ready with pricing and be confident in stating it. Better yet, show the value of what you offer with data and statistics. Additionally, assure the company you carry insurance, have a liability waiver that includes the company, and insist on a contract. Your contract should state your employment status as an independent contractor, the length of the contract or program, and your compensation rate.

Additionally, there are companies that corporations and businesses work with to create and manage their employee wellness programs. Not all companies will hire you independently, especially the major corporations like Google and Facebook, for example. Wellness management companies function similarly to employment agencies, you apply to the agency, not directly to the business itself. Businesses in need of yoga teachers or wellness programs contact the management companies, and they contract you as the teacher. The downside is they take a cut and you won't earn as much as you could if hired directly. If you'd like to explore this route, look up local employee fitness or wellness management solution companies. They are a bit tricky to find, as the wording to describe such a company isn't universal, so play with different terms in your searches. Here are two examples to help you get started:

- BeneFitness (currently in Portland, Oregon, USA): www.benefitnesslife.com
- Innergy Corporate Yoga (all over Canada): www.innergycorporateyoga.com

Teach Athletes

This may not be everyone's cup of tea or niche, but yoga for athletes is definitely on the rise. As athletes look for ways to gain a competitive edge over their opponents, yoga is coming forth as the latest weapon. Creating flexibility, preventing injury, increasing range of motion, and improving mental focus are just some of the benefits athletes are loving.

Within athletics, the opportunities reach far and wide. You can work with kids or adults, schools or universities, individual athletes or teams, clubs and camps, trainers and coaches, fitness facilities or gyms, recreational leagues and more. Like corporate gigs, with athletes you want to be professional, approach them with programming, and acquire a contract. You can also propose a similar compensation rate that will increase with the number of team members or participants.

I should mention, working with athletes is different than teaching a general public class. You need to understand what that specific group needs. What are the repetitive movements and problems areas of the body specific to that sport? Consider if the athlete is in the off-season or game season, and how much physical load is already being demanded of their body. Usually, athletes train hard enough as it is, and as much as they may want a sweaty, tough yoga practice, what they really need is a calming, noncompetitive practice. A big challenge with athletes is creating an environment where they understand and respect that there is no winning in yoga and it's not about the external form. If this is route you want to explore, look up a teacher training for working with athletes and check out Sage Rountree's books and trainings (www.sagerountree.com).

Teach Skype Classes

As someone who is scared to be in front of the camera, I'll admit I've never taught a Skype class, and I know this option won't appeal to everyone. We've got to be authentic to ourselves. However, there's something to be said for stepping out of your comfort zone and exploring new things. For some teachers being in front of the camera is their comfort zone. Remember Jen from the opening story? Jen had a background in acting, so taking her career to the camera was a natural step. If you are one of those people or are willing to try something new, Skype classes are an awesome way to reach people from all corners of the globe, especially those who don't feel comfortable in studios or don't have the time. As small as you may think your niche may be, it'll become a whole lot bigger when you expand your population pool from your local community to the world abroad.

Become A Coach

The life of a yogi involves much more than the asana practice. As a yoga, health or wellness coach, you can help students take their yoga practice off the mat and turn it into a lifestyle. Talk about making a difference in someone's life! As a coach you can help people beyond the physical practice with spiritual teachings, healthy habits, and emotional support. It's the perfect way to integrate your Ayurveda training, nutrition knowledge, counseling background, understanding of The Yoga Sutras and love for green juice.

Do your students ever tell you they struggle to get to their mat as often as they wish or they want to learn more about the spiritual side of yoga? This is the perfect opportunity to step in as a coach. Not only does a coach provide the knowledge and resources to help people achieve their desires, but coaches are there for accountability. This is often the one thing people need most - to be held to their goals and what they set out to do. It's really rewarding and impactful work, and just so happens to be very lucrative as well.

Coaching rates can range between $75 and $250 an hour, and the role comes with a ton of flexibility. You can work from anywhere because coaching doesn't have to be done in-person; much of it is done via email, phone and Skype. You can also switch up traditional one-on-one coaching with small group coaching and online programs. In those situations, it's usually not an hourly rate, but a flat fee for the program. Whatever you choose to do in the realm of coaching, be legit with it. If you're going to offer Ayurveda guidance, educate yourself with formal training. You'll also want to get proper coaching training yourself. There are loads of certifications out there, so do some thorough research before choosing a certification program. Here are a couple:

- Health Coach with Institute of Integrative Nutrition: www.integrativenutrition.com
- Health Coach Institute: www.healthcoachinstitute.com
- Yoga Health Coaching: www.yogahealthcoaching.com

- Nutritional Therapy Association: www.nutritionaltherapy.com

Facilitate Retreats

It can be daunting to think about organizing an oversees retreat if you've never done it before. However, retreats don't have to be in far-off exotic locations. Due to travel expenses, I've heard from experienced teachers that a local retreat can easily boast the same profit margin as a high-end destination retreat. When thinking about a local retreat, consider first where you live. You might already live in a desirable place. Do you live near the beach, on a rustic ranch, in the mountains or in a major metropolitan city like Houston, New York or San Francisco? Consider, anywhere in the U.S. could be a destination retreat for people from other countries and vice versa. If you live in say, Europe, Australia or Asia, your hometown can be a cost-effective place to host a destination retreat for foreigners.

When organizing a retreat close to where you live, look for a unique bed and breakfast, a quaint lodge, a hot springs resort, a temple or spiritual center, a relaxing spa, or a local retreat center like the Mount Madonna Center in California (www.mountmadonna.org). Consider partnering up with other healers and teachers to co-host a retreat and assume some of the responsibility. Attend other local retreats to experience it from the participant side, get some ideas and figure out what you like and don't like. If you don't know what to charge, research like retreats to see what similar rates are. Of course, make sure your price covers all of your costs and turns a profit. Like workshops, retreat income comes in lump sums, so many teachers set it aside for saving instead of depending on it for monthly income.

Kundalini Yoga teacher, Charanpal Kaur, says international retreats are all about "collaboration and community" (www.charanpalmusic.com). When planning an international retreat, Charanpal advises teachers to find someone in the local community who speaks the language and has connections. Look at what your travel costs are, and negotiate a contract that will ensure your minimum expenses will be covered.

Leader of Align & Shine women's retreat in Costa Rica and co-founder of Resilient Leadership Retreats for veterans, Sarah Plummer Taylor knows a lot about planning retreats (www.sempersarah.com). Sarah explains, "Picking a facility you've actually been to is key. Don't go sight unseen." Sarah once booked a retreat at a venue she'd never been to and found herself apologizing to her attendees over and over because the venue was much more rugged than what the facility portrayed online.

Sarah's second piece of advice is to, "Build out a team where you can. Even if you're the best yoga teacher, maybe people don't want to take 10 classes from you in a week. I like variety, so I bring in other teachers. It also builds in a team environment that translates to the attendees as well, getting to know one another and getting closer". If Sarah personally knows a teacher who will be in attendance, she'll even invite them to guest teach at her retreat as a fun option to enhance the experience for everyone. Sarah also hires a photographer (sometimes on barter, sometimes paid) to capture the retreat. For attendees, this adds a lot of value as people love to share the images and look back on special moments. For Sarah, it adds value to her business because she can use these photos for future marketing.

Lastly, Sarah recommends, "Take some of the work out of it over time by repeating the venue space. This goes back to relationship building. If you build relationships with the people who work there from the front office staff to the chefs to the cleaners, you know them well and planning gets easier each time".

If you'd love to plan a retreat, but have no experience in doing so, a company like Trip Tribe can be very helpful with organizing it (https://triptribe.com/). These businesses take care of securing a venue, booking management, food menus, payments and much more. Be a bit cautious, however, I've heard mixed reviews from teachers about their satisfaction with such businesses. Do your research, read reviews, and ask a ton of questions. You may even want to reach out to teachers who have used the company you're interested in before and ask for their feedback.

Yoga Journal has published a 3-part series of articles written by Jodi Mardesich to assist teachers in their retreat planning. Check them out:

- Beyond The Studio: Retreats Part I: www.yogajournal.com/article/teach/beyond-the-studio-retreats-part-i

- Yoga Retreats: Part II: www.yogajournal.com/article/teach/yoga-retreats-part-ii
- Sell Out Your Yoga Retreat: Part III: www.yogajournal.com/article/teach/yoga-retreats-part-iii

Go On Tour

A tour is especially great for teachers who love to travel or those who have a large social media following abroad. Bilingual yoga teacher, Yely Staley, always knew she wanted to bring yoga to Hispanic and Latin communities (www.yogayely.com). Over Instagram, she built connections with teachers and studios in Argentina and Chile that transformed into teaching invitations and an international tour.

Like Yely, with some networking and outreach efforts, you can book a teaching tour for yourself. As a guest teacher, you can tour your home city, state, country and abroad. It's a great opportunity to put your second language or niche to work by teaching specialized classes not generally offered in studios.

For a passionate traveler and yoga teacher, what's not to like about going on tour? In addition, check out Yoga Trade for unique teaching opportunities around the globe (www.yogatrade.com) that can help as you book out your tour.

Host Webinars

Short for web-based seminar, a webinar is a presentation, lecture, or workshop that is transmitted over the internet using video conferencing software. What makes a webinar different than other forms of online video, such as downloadable classes or lectures, is that webinars are interactive and done in real-time. The presenter can interact with participants, participants can interact with each other, and participants can interact with the presenter. Webinars also differ from pre-recorded video presentations because they are live and thus, they are active income that depends on your direct time. But don't let that stop you. Because of the ability to interact, it's easier to make connections and strengthen your relationships, which significantly impacts your brand and following.

Think of webinars like virtual workshops that allow you to reach beyond one location. They are super convenient, as neither you nor the participant need to leave their own home, and are more cost-effective because you don't have to share the revenue with a studio. One webinar a month could equate to a substantial amount of income. For example, if you charged $20 for a 90-minute webinar on the Yoga Sutras of Patanjali and were able to get 50 registered participants, you could earn an extra $1,000 a month!

Webinar software is widely available with a simple Google search, but here are a two to get you started:

- WebinarJam (www.webinarjam.com)
- GoToMeeting (www.gotomeeting.com)

Teach at A Local College

Colleges and universities offer yoga in their gyms, but also as semester classes. Look up the colleges in your area and visit their course catalog to see if they offer yoga for semester credits. If they don't already offer yoga, propose a course to the respective administration staff. If they already do, inquire if there's an opening to assist, substitute or add another course. Colleges like the College of San Mateo in California even offer a full 200 hour yoga teacher training program, yielding yet another opportunity for you to broaden your teaching horizons and income streams (www.collegeofsanmateo.edu/yoga/degrees_yoga_cs.asp).

Teach at K-12 Schools

As yoga grows in popularity and the benefits become more well-known, academic institutions of all shapes and sizes are integrating yoga programs, not just colleges. I've seen programs in all sectors from public to private to charter, and in elementary, middle and high schools. In developing your program, you could build it out as a two-week physical education unit, a full semester elective or a short to long term after school program. But first, get to know the school and design your program based on their needs. It might be centered on movement, exercise and the physical benefits of yoga, or you could focus your program on social-emotional learning and leadership development. If this excites you, but you don't know where to begin, you can get involved with an established organization, such as Spirit Of Youth Yoga who licenses their curriculum and contracts instructors (www.spiritofyouthyoga.com). Additionally, here's an evidence-based article full of information on the topic: Implementing Yoga Within The School Curriculum (www.emeraldinsight.com/doi/abs/10.1108/JCS-10-2014-0044).

Partner with Like Businesses

The options are endless when it comes to partnering up with other businesses in your niche. One of my favorite partnerships I created as a studio owner was with a non-profit community farm called Veggielution (www.veggielution.org). During spring and summer months, we offered donation-based yoga in the farm fresh air. It was a great opportunity to cross promote with a like-minded organization and offer something unique to our community. Plus, as the program grew and gained exposure, it led us to other beneficial community partnerships.

Consider your niche and find other businesses where you can offer weekly or monthly classes. For example, you could offer yoga for back pain at a chiropractic office or story-time yoga at a children's museum. The key component to building partnerships is networking and meeting representatives from other businesses. Look up meetings for small businesses in your area, as well as meetups and niche specific networking events. I know it can be intimidating and easy to create a ton of excuses why it won't be worth your time, but believe me, they're worth it. I used to try to talk myself out of it, but then I'd meet the owner of an apartment complex who let me put private yoga flyers up in her lobby or the owner of a coffee shop who opened up his shop as a place for me to teach to his staff and customers. You never know who you're going to meet and what door may open up. Networking is crucial in the beginning phases of building your business.

Speaking Engagements, Festivals & Expos

This is another avenue where having a niche comes in handy. When you're recognized as an expert in your niche, you open yourself up to opportunities to speak at expos, summits and symposiums. These can be online or in-person events. Today, companies from Yoga International to Hay House Publishing are pulling together teachers from around the globe for online summits and conferences. Once you've established a small following with social media and/or an email list, you can collaborate with other teachers and healers to offer a group online symposium. These are excellent opportunities to grow your brand, following, expertise and bank account. When first starting out, you may need to speak at a number of small events for free, but eventually you can bring in substantial earnings from speaking engagements.

Remember Courtney Mitchell from earlier in the book? She's the co-founder of The Yoga Expo (www.theyogaexpo.org), an all-day yoga event showcasing local teachers and vendors that tours around the United States. Peruse the websites of such events and look for a link (sometimes in the website's footer) to "participate" or send them an email through the contact form. See what's around your city, and remember it doesn't have to be yoga specific, but it should relate to your niche.

Teaching at festivals can be a similar experience, yielding comparable benefits. Festivals are popping up left and right from large ones that appeal to the masses, to small community one-day events. Keep your eyes out and don't be afraid to reach out to the organizers of such events and offer your expertise. It takes time to elevate yourself to a point where people invite you, and chances are you're missing opportunities if you just sit back and wait for things to come to you.

Certify or Train Teachers

Another great opportunity to put your niche to work is by teaching other instructors how to work within your niche population. A 15-30 hour specialty certification or training program can generate between $150-$500 (sometimes more) in revenue per participant. Create a signature training that's repeatable and host it as often as you like. It's a great way to build your brand and expertise, while serving as a means to scale your business. Once teachers have gone through you training, you can invite them into your team as you grow.

Forewarning, examine your niche carefully to determine if there's room and a need for more teachers. Don't create competition for yourself, especially in your local area if there's not substantial room for growth. On the other hand, I don't want you avoid scaling your business for fear of competition. With enough time and experience in any niche, you'll know whether or not there's room for more teachers, so don't rush this option.

Hire A Team of Instructors

This option can be considered both active and passive income, but the general idea is to scale your business to a point where you can hire a team of instructors to staff private classes and events. Let's say you specialize in wedding day yoga for brides, couples and wedding parties. As you grow your business, you can staff wedding day classes with other instructors who you've hired as independent contractors. For some of you, maybe you'll want to build your business with this type of scalability in mind from the beginning. For others, once the momentum is really going, you might find you simply can't fill the demand alone and hire staff out of necessity. Either way, while generating revenue for your business you're giving other teachers an additional source of income. #awesome

PASSIVE INCOME

Remember, passive income is pay that does not require a direct exchange of your time for money. Passive income streams can make you money while you sleep. However, many forms of passive income entail upfront time to create and setup, but the important part to understand is that by comparison, it involves very little time to maintain. A classic example, although quickly being replaced by the internet, is the yoga DVD. Making a DVD took time for a yoga teacher to plan and bring to market, but once it became available to the public, the DVD could generate revenue any time of day or night, while requiring less and less time to maintain as time goes on.

The internet has done a great deal for passive income opportunities. Take the yoga DVD. A teacher would have to invest a large upfront cost in order to produce, stock and deliver the product. With the internet, now that same video content can be delivered without the high cost of producing the tangible DVD itself and shipping it to the consumer.

Before we get into passive (and digital) income streams, I have to preface this by telling you all these approaches require some form of an existing audience. Said differently, when selling digital products, you've got to have a network of people to sell your product to. The internet can be a crowded space and a tricky place to be seen. It's not an "if you build it, they will come" type of situation. But don't worry, I've got you covered in the Mindful Marketing chapter. When you read through these options, just know that I'll help you grow a community to share your products with.

Create A Virtual Studio

It's true, when teaching online you are much more removed from your students than teaching in person, but there are so many benefits that it's worth a deeper look. Just about every industry and business is already serving their audience online in some shape or form because the demand is there and people want it. As I've mentioned before, many folks around the globe who are interested in yoga will never set foot in a traditional studio and for countless reasons, such as these:

- They're intimidated by the yogi stereotype and fear they won't fit in
- They can't find classes that suit their unique needs or body types at a studio
- There is no studio in their town
- They don't have transportation to get to the studio
- They don't have the time it takes to travel to and from the studio
- They can't afford studio pricing
- They don't have anyone to stay home with their kids
- The studio class times don't work with their schedule
- The instructors aren't trained or equipped to accommodate their special condition, needs or limitation

As you can gather, bringing your teaching online makes yoga more accessible, positions you to meet people where they are, and enables you to serve those who aren't currently being served by the traditional studio. A virtual studio delivers the convenience of yoga anytime, anywhere to your students in a way that a brick-and-mortar studio simply can't. You can offer a variety of class durations, skill levels, styles and themes to work within your niche and reach people internationally. You can literally bring your teachings to homes in the farthest corners of the world. Your reach becomes limitless with online teaching.

When building out your virtual studio, you have a ton of room for flexibility, creativity, freedom and earning potential. Depending on how you'd like to build it out, people can purchase classes a la carte, as packages or as a monthly membership. It's truly teaching on your terms. You teach where you want, when you want and how you want to. You choose your own pricing structure and you generate profit for yourself instead of someone else's business. Like the limitless reach of a virtual studio, the amount you can earn is unlimited and entirely up to you.

Another advantage to bringing your teachings online, is that you can easily incorporate your other passions and modalities. Say you also have a background in nutrition and want to help folks live healthier, happier lives. In addition to yoga classes that could be focused on weight loss and detoxing, you can offer self-acceptance meditations and weekly juice or meal recipes. It's an amazing way to help people holistically and have a greater impact through your own comprehensive programs.

Once you have your studio built out with some basic offerings, the magic starts to happen. Without any limitations on your hours of operation, your online studio is open and working for you 24/7, and you don't even have to be there. In a Yoga Journal article by Sage Rountree, Sadie Nardini shared this insight about teaching online, "For the same energy expenditure it takes me to teach one class, people can experience it again and again, in wildly different times and places. It's a dream come true to be able to show up for all of them without compromising the quality of my energy or my teachings" (www.yogajournal.com/article/teach/lights-camera-yoga).

It must be said, however, that even with the vast opportunities a virtual studio affords, you have to be ok with spending a fair amount of time at your computer. You'll need to edit your videos, update your website, grow your following with social media, blog, and be an active member in your niche's online community. There's no getting around it, a virtual studio requires computer time and some technical skills, but don't worry, the technical stuff can easily be learned with a friend's help, YouTube tutorials, and patience. If the thought of working at a computer sounds daunting, think about this: with an online business, your office can be anywhere and your working hours can be any time of the day. You can take off to Thailand and work from a bungalow on the beach, you can tag along while your spouse travels for work, and you can easily step away from the laptop to pick up a sick child from school. It's your studio, your business, and your freedom. From your branding to the actual content you offer, your studio is a reflection of who you are and your style of teaching.

Let's get back to the technical stuff and constructing your studio. There are multiple platforms out there to support your new venture. Starting with the most basic, YouTube is a free distribution platform that's super easy to use. Your website is where people will learn about your classes and offerings, but YouTube is where the videos will be stored. In order to make your videos available for purchase, you'll need to make them private instead of public, so only people who've paid can watch. Your payment system will also integrate with your website, which will in turn give access to your videos. The hang-up here (and this may change in the future) is that currently YouTube requires that you already have a channel with at least 1,000 subscribers for paid content. So, that means offering free videos until you have enough subscribers to offer paid content. For more information about setting up paid content with YouTube, visit https://support.google.com/youtube/answer/324912 7?hl=en&ref_topic=3249164.

Moving up a level from YouTube, the other options I'd like to share with you are PowHow (www.powhow.com/open-your-own-studio) and Namastream (www.namastream.com). PowHow is website designed to host and sell online classes based in fitness, art and music. Powhow manages all software, videos, and hosting for a monthly fee between $15-$20. Check out Sadie Nardini's online studio (www.powhow.com/classes/sadie-nardinisrockin-online-yoga-studio). Sadie has a variety of offerings from single class videos for $5 to an $8 monthly subscription to themed packages for $19.99.

Namastream has a higher price point, but it's much more robust and built out specifically for yoga and wellness studios. Namastream's pricing varies according to your needs for storage space, quantity of student accounts and whether you sign-up for a monthly or annual plan. Plans currently range from $79 - $179 per month. They provide tremendous support to help you along the way with resources such as a free Gear Guide, a Facebook group, an advice blog, and private consulting.

Sell Online Courses

Very similar to having a virtual studio, creating and selling online courses boasts many of the same benefits and freedom. Online courses can be signature offerings within your virtual studio or they can stand alone as a component of your business. Although the word "course" has an academic tone to it, think of it instead like an online workshop or series. Like a workshop, a course setting gives you the time and space to dive deep into yogic teachings. A course is essentially a series of lessons on a particular topic strung together in sequential order, and another opportunity to ignite your creative soul. The content of your course can consist of videos, audio, slideshows, worksheets, PDFs, digital books and more. Businesses and teachers around the world are recognizing the strength of online courses to deepen yogic studies, just take a look at Yoga International's array of online courses (www.yogainternational.com/ecourses).

Again, Sadie Nardini has paved the way as well. In addition to Sadie's virtual studio, she sells online courses via another popular platform called Udemy. Seane Corn also uses Udemy to host her online course, The Yoga Of Awakening. Udemy is a decent platform for selling courses, and popular because it was one of the first ones. However, online learning has grown so much that we have hundreds of options now more adept to serve the independent teacher building an online component of their business. Here's a few reasons why I don't recommend Udemy:

1. It's a marketplace, so your course will be competing with all the other like courses within Udemy.

2. You don't have full control over your course. You can't price your course for more than $50 and once it's up on Udemy, you don't have the option to take it down.

3. Udemy prohibits teachers from transferring students into their own communication and email lists. They require you to stay within Udemy's internal messaging system. That means when you sell a course to someone via Udemy, you can't add them to your newsletter and notify them when you have new offerings, which you definitely want to be able to do.

Instead, I recommend using Teachable (www.teachable.com). As opposed to competing in a marketplace like Udemy, you can create your own marketplace of online courses and programs. With Teachable, you can customize your courses with your personal branding and easily import videos, PDFs, and other content while Teachable takes care of hosting, sign-ups and payments. Pricing plans depend on your volume needs and will currently run you between $39 and $99 a month, but the features are worth every penny. The system supports multiple languages, is fully optimized for web or mobile, comes equipped with learning tools such as quizzes, discussion forums, and student surveys, and they provide comprehensive analytics on your course data.

If you're interested in creating a simple video course without a ton of supplemental content or features such as discussion forums, you could use another platform for selling your courses called Gumroad (www.gumraod.com) for only $10 a month plus a small percentage of each sale.

A couple of other things to consider when creating online courses:

- Will your course have open or closed enrollment? Open enrollment lets participants register any ol' day of the year, while closed enrollment means participants can only register when you specify the course is being offered. Each option has its pros and cons. For example, open enrollment brings in money all year long, but then again, when people know they can enroll anytime they tend to put it off for another day that often never comes. With closed enrollment, you may choose to only offer your course twice a year which builds in limitation and a need to act now instead of perpetually putting it off. Additionally, if your course entails personal engagement with you, such as coaching calls or group Facebook discussions, then closed enrollment could be more ideal because your time will only be required a few times a year, during your specified time.

- Will participants have access to all the course content immediately, or will it drip out in a timed release format? For example, say you have a six-month course. You could release the entire course all at once and let participants move through it on their own, or you could drip out the content in timely intervals over the six months. Most experts in online learning suggest that dripping out the content is best because each time you send out a new module, it reminds people of the course and helps keep them on track and engaged. Then, for the occasional person who wants it all at once, you can make the exception. However, you have to decide what is best for you and your course.

If this is a road you'd like to travel, before you start designing your course listen to episode *218: Starting An Online Course? Best Practices & Getting People To Follow Through* of the Smart Passive Income Podcast with Pat Flynn and Ankur Nagpal (the founder of Teachable).

Audible Yoga

Audible Yoga is a great platform to create passive income or support yourself as a traveling yoga teacher (www.audibleyoga.com). Yogis from all over the world can join Audible Yoga with a monthly membership that allows them to take audio classes anytime, anywhere, while the teachers who lead the classes earn commissions on downloads. All you need is an app and a headset to earn extra money on the classes you're already teaching.

Allie Lehnhardt is a yoga teacher and military wife who has moved over 13 times (www.facebook.com/Allie-Cat-Yoga-LLC-Audible-Yoga-Teacher-Code-11978). She's a brilliant example of a teacher who has taken responsibility for the direction of her career. Dispersing her eggs into multiple baskets, Allie makes use of active and passive income streams with private, corporate, military and audio classes. "Being in the military", Allie said, "you have to embrace change and uncertainty. Your next best friend isn't going to knock on your door. As in life, you have to go out and seek your own opportunities", just as she is doing with her career.

For Allie, Audible Yoga is not only a means of passive income, but a way for students to continue practicing with her, regardless of where she's currently living. Allie simply records her public classes and uploads them to her Audible Yoga profile. Once her classes are available, the students Allie personally refers to the platform can download her classes, just as students already using the platform can discover her and take her classes. For each download Allie earns a commission, as well as for each monthly subscriber she refers.

When I asked Allie about the benefits of audio only and no video, she explained that students enjoy the simplicity of the audio format. Without the need to look at a screen and compare oneself to who's on the screen, audio gives the student an opportunity to connect with their own body and experience.

Additionally, the audio format eliminates the time-consuming process of production that comes with video. It's a great option for teachers who want to bring their classes online, but are camera shy like me.

Write an eBook

The publishing world has changed dramatically with internet advances and the introduction of Amazon's Kindle. Now, even bestselling authors stand to earn substantially more by forgoing conventional contract publishing and opting to self-publish. With this flourishing landscape of digital reading and independent authors, Amazon now sells more eBooks than printed books, according to their 2011 press release (http://phx.corporate-ir.net/phoenix.zhtml?c=176060&p=irol-newsArticle&ID=1565581&highlight).

Take a look at any book genre or industry and you'll no doubt find a plethora of eBooks covering a range of interests and topics from science fiction to dog training to auto mechanics, and yoga is no exception. A simple search in Amazon for yoga eBooks will give you an idea for what's out there, but don't be intimidated by the search results. There is still plenty of room in the market, and you'll have your own niche and unique audience interested in what you have to say.

As with most business ideas, your first step is market research. Spend some time browsing the top eBooks on Amazon in your niche and get an idea for what's already being done and what's lacking. Read the reviews and find out what people like about the books and where they're falling short. You want to get an intuitive feel for the market, what's selling, what isn't and why. Moreover, figure out where can you fill a gap and carve out a space for your unique voice and message.

Once you've nailed down your angle and niche, start with an outline and continue through the writing process. When it comes time to publish, you have two main choices to distribute and sell your book. The first option is to sell within a marketplace like Amazon. With Amazon's Kindle Direct Publishing (KDP), the process is very simple (www.kdp.amazon.com). KDP seamlessly converts your book from a Microsoft Word document (or other various formats) into a Kindle eBook format.

For your cover, you can go DIY style with KDP's cover creator tool, Photoshop or Canva (www.canva.com). If you want to go the professional route, I suggest hiring a designer from Fivrr (www.fiverr.com) or 99Designs (ww.99designs.com).

The second option to sell your book is on your own website. With this option, your book format will be a PDF, as the Kindle format is strictly for Amazon. If choosing the website option, you'll simply convert your Microsoft Word document into a PDF and deliver it to the buyer via email (either with your email marketing service such as MailChimp (www.mailchimp.com) or a commerce service such as Gumroad (www.gumroad.com).

Both options come with advantages and disadvantages. To start, if you decide to publish with KDP, then you will be competing within the Amazon marketplace with other like books. At the same time, being on Amazon can give you exposure to millions of potential buyers. However, there's a number of factors that contribute as to whether or not Amazon actually puts your book in front of potential buyers, so you'll need to learn the basics of optimizing to sell on Amazon. For more on optimization read this

article from SemRush.com
(https://www.semrush.com/blog/amazon-seo-tactics-because-amazon-is-a-search-engine-too/).

Another cool thing about publishing with KDP is that Amazon has another platform called CreateSpace that allows people to buy print copies of your book (www.createspace.com). Without having to stock inventory of your book, CreateSpace will print your book one at a time, as each order is placed and ship it directly to the buyer. Pretty dang sweet if you ask me!

But then again, we have another disadvantage to publishing with Amazon: limitations on pricing your eBook. In order for them to maintain their dominant position in online book sales, they have to keep their pricing competitive. For a self-publishing author, that means Amazon has a tricky way of steering you into their ideal price range of $2.99-$9.99. If you price your book within that range, Amazon will take 30% of each sale for their part in the process. However, if you choose to price your book above $9.99, Amazon takes an astronomical 70% of each sale. So, what do authors do? They either keep their price under $9.99 or sell their books independently through their own website in PDF format.

Choosing to publish your eBook as a PDF and selling it directly on your website gives you a ton of freedom in pricing and distribution. But, as I've touched upon, it's then completely on you to promote and sell the book (which is definitely doable with some know-how). Therefore, the decision to sell on your website and/or Amazon becomes a decision of weighing the pros and cons against your goals and experience. Do you already have a substantial audience to sell to or do you need to take advantage of Amazon's exposure and reach? Is this your first book? Are you already established in your niche? Again, do some of you own research on creating and selling eBooks to come to your own conclusion of what will work best for you. I wish I could give you a solid answer, but there is no universal direction. What works for some doesn't work for others, but at least now you have a starting point.

For a complete guide to writing and publishing an eBook, passive income expert Pat Flynn has you covered with his FREE download, eBooks The Smart Way
(www.smartpassiveincome.com/ebooks-the-smart-way).

Monetize A Blog or YouTube Channel

Blogging and offering free YouTube videos are both methods of building your audience while providing valuable content to folks. Simultaneously, these platforms can also generate revenue through advertisements.

Hold up, did she just say advertisements!? Yep, I know the thought makes many of you cringe, but it's a viable option to consider should you be open to it.

Yeah it sucks having to watch a Ford commercial before the cute video of puppies falling off couches, but what if you think about it in a different light? That advertisement may very well be an important line of income for the video creator and what enables them to continue creating free videos. Most people won't mind sitting through a commercial for a free morning yoga practice that starts their day off right. The same goes for blogging. Placing ads on a blog page is one of the primary strategies bloggers use to generate income from what they do and all the free content they put out. If you already have a blog or have been thinking about starting one, monetizing it through advertisements is something to consider and do some research on.

Write Articles for Publications or Studios

This is a really fun option to earn some extra bucks if you love writing. I can personally say it's thrilling to see a piece I've written published through a game-changing organization like Yoga International. With the amount of content large publications need to produce for their websites and social media handles, it's also easier than you might think to get published.

Unfortunately, most of the major publications in the yoga world don't pay contributing authors. I hope this changes in the future, but at the moment, the only one I know that pays is Yoga International. For each accepted article, Yoga International pays the author a minimum of $50 with the potential to earn up to $200 (https://yogainternational.com/article/view/write-or-teach-for-yoga-international).

Rest assured, there are other options and you aren't restricted to only yoga publications:

- T'AI CHI Magazine focuses on martial arts, health, meditation and spiritual growth and pays $75-$500 per article (http://tai-chi.com/index.php/writers-guidelines).
- Earth Island Journal covers environmental and animal rights topics (I know many of you are vegetarians) and pays $0.25 a word (http://www.earthisland.org/journal/index.php/guidelines/).
- Radish Magazine centers on healthy eating, but also dives into the "body, mind & soul" category and pays $50-$150 per article (http://radishmagazine.com/guidelines).
- Wellbeing Magazine focuses on natural therapies, caring for animals, exercise and natural beauty and pays $100-$500 per article (https://www.wellbeing.com.au/contribute).

Be sure to also look up publications in your niche and submit related articles.

Studios also have a need for writers. Blogging can play an important role in boosting a studio's Google rankings, but the owners often don't have the time to write consistent blog posts. This creates an opportunity for teachers like you to contribute to the success of a studio, while contributing to your bank account. Before proposing this idea to a studio owner, make sure you understand the basics of blogging and SEO (search engine optimization). Here's a good introductory article to business blogging http://blog.hubspot.com/marketing/the-benefits-of-business-blogging.

Lastly, you can also try writing for a local newspaper or magazine. You can find independent publications based on lifestyle, family, athletics, food, beauty, arts, culture, events, etc., many of which have a "health" or "wellness" section or column.

GATHER YOUR IDEAS

Start with a simple brainstorm. List out everything that comes to mind as a possible way to offer your services to your niche. Where could you teach? How could you deliver yoga classes to your niche? What businesses could you partner with? How can you meet people where they are? Let the pen flow and don't shy from writing something down regardless of how off the wall or intimidating it may sound in your head. Each niche is different, so be creative and think outside the box.

Say you're interested in prenatal yoga and working with mothers, your brainstorm list might look something like this:

- In-person private classes for pregnant women
- Prenatal Skype classes for women around the world
- Group classes for local moms clubs
- Weekly prenatal classes at a nearby birthing center
- A class series to prepare the body for natural childbirth at a community center (or partnering with a birthing center or chiropractic office)
- Published articles in parenting magazines and online publications
- An online self-care course for busy moms
- A postnatal online course for new moms
- A virtual studio for mothers featuring classes, meditations, and healthy meal recipes
- An eBook for mindful parenting
- An annual self-care retreat for mothers with a partner business/organization/teacher

- Teaching or speaking at the BirthWorks Conference
- Hosting a seminar or exhibiting at the Natural Family Expo
- A monthly class for moms and kids at a local children's museum
- A membership site for mothers featuring a daily Q&A, a weekly video class, an advice blog, and a monthly webinar

CHAPTER 5:
BUSINESS PLANNING

"Vision without action is just a dream. Action without vision just passes the time. Vision with action can change the world." – Joel A. Barker

You've made it this far because you aren't just another dreamer. You're willing to explore new terrain and face the challenge of taking the reins. Now it's time to pull your vision into a plan of actionable steps to realization. As Tony Robbins says, "Knowledge is not power. Knowledge is only potential power. Action is power".

A business plan tells the story of your business. It represents your current position, your vision, and your plans for realizing that vision. Like Pada Bandha, a business plan provides a stable foundation from which to build upon, and is essential to being successful. Unless you need financial assistance starting your business, you don't have worry about sharing your business plan with anyone else. It's your personal roadmap.

A business plan answers the following questions:

- What is your business idea or what is your existing business?
- What is your vision for this business?
- Who are your ideal clients and what motivates them to choose you?
- How will you reach clients to let them know about your business?
- How will you stand out in the crowd and differentiate yourself from your competitors?
- What is your financial overview? How much will it cost you to run your business and how much money will you make?

ANATOMY OF A BUSINESS PLAN

Remember, your business plan is your personal roadmap. **It outlines the path you intend to take to get from A to B, and it serves as a guide should you lose your way or come across an obstacle.** It helps you connect the dots and bring all your ideas together into one convenient place, so don't skip this step. After all, if you don't take the time to put together the pieces, you'll never get to the big picture.

Here's what your plan should include (you can think of this in terms of the 5 Ws):

1. **Executive Summary** (the WHY): In a nutshell, this presents your vision, values and mission. Think about why your business does what it does. I find the most important part here is identifying your business values because they serve as the base that supports all your business decisions and actions. When you're unsure of something, refer to your values, align with them and act accordingly.

2. **Target Market** (the WHO): This is a deep understanding of who you are going to serve, and details your market research. It identifies your ideal client and describes their demographic and characteristics. Most importantly, this section outlines what their primary needs are based on real data, not just what you think they need.

3. **Services** (the WHAT): Precisely, what does your business offer and what are you helping your target audience with? Here's a hint, it's not just yoga. You offer a piece of mind, a

body free of pain, the ability to play and keep up with one's grandchildren, or the chance for your student to beat their buddies in golf. In whatever shape or form, your services start with offering a better life. After you've gotten very clear on the WHAT, then break it down even further into your actual services (corporate gigs, private clients, online classes, etc.).

4. **Marketing Plan** (the HOW): How will you reach people and how will they learn of your business? What lines of communication will you use, and what will your branding look like? Moreover, how will you present your message to your target audience in a way they can relate to?

5. **Operations** (the WHERE, WHEN & more): This section outlines your perfect schedule (when you actually want to be teaching/working - what days and times) and where you'll be holding classes (home studio, partner business, community center, online, etc.). It also describes how you're actually going to run your business and execute basic functions. What technology will support your business such as a website provider, an email marketing service, a payment system, etc.

This could also include any equipment you need to run your business, such as yoga mats and video gear. Additionally, it can be viewed as a checklist, ensuring legal forms such as waivers are in place, your insurance policy is up to date, you have a business bank account, you've formed a legal entity if need be and you've acquired any necessary business licenses, etc.

6. **Financial Plan**: What's your current financial situation and where would you like your business to bring you? What are your financial goals and how will you get there? Based on your services, business expenses and ideal schedule, how many classes do you need to teach or how many online courses do you need to sell? How will you keep track of your income and expenses? What will be your bookkeeping method?

7. **Future Development**: Wrap it up by defining business milestones you intend to reach. This can include financial milestones or milestones in your reach, as with email subscribers or the number of private clients you have on the books. What are your big picture and long-term goals- 1 year, 5 years, and 10 years?

You may have a lot of this done by now, or at least mapped out from previous sections of the book. If you've already crafted your trademark story, have a niche in mind and have done some thorough market research, then pulling your ideas together into a business plan will likely be easy with just a few blanks to fill in. Otherwise, **let it be a process as you unearth the possibilities and discover your path**. Move through it stage by stage and let it be a writing exercise that helps extract your thoughts and desires, and assists in shaping your business.

If you're still unsure of who you want to work with, go back to Chapter 3 and get in touch with your personal "why"- the reason why you teach yoga. What transformation did you experience that made you want to teach? Think back to that defining moment and think about the position or circumstance you were in. Who else (as in what group, community or demographic of people) is in the same boat as you once were?

If you just can't seem to figure out a unique offering and niche for your business, then I suggest you stick with your day job for now, and start teaching different types of people and exposing yourself to new teaching environments. Teach at a hospital, work with kids, pick up an athlete private client, and try on as many different hats as you can. Like Goldilocks, taste the cold porridge and then taste the hot porridge, and maybe you'll discover the warm porridge that's just right for you.

CHAPTER 6:
MINDFUL MARKETING

Marketing is about selling and promoting, both of which tend to make yoga teachers queasy. However, when you view selling as helping, the fear of being a sleazy car salesman subsides. Realize, we're not in the business of selling yoga, we're in the business of creating change. From this point of view, **it's not about the money - it's about providing massive value**. When you're all about the money, your approach to sales is all about benefitting yourself, as opposed to helping someone solve a problem or overcome a challenge. If you promote and sell from the intention of helping, you'll experience gratifying success and the money will follow. Your earnings are simply a byproduct of how well you help your community.

If marketing scares you, here's a trick to overcome what holds so many teachers back. If you view promoting your business as self-promotion, then it will be just that - self-promotion. Why you ask? Because when you put yourself on center stage and focus on What-I-Do, then it becomes all about you and not your message. With you at the center of what you're selling, the fear of rejection often arises and scares people off. But remember, it's not about you. It's about those who you serve. Your clients are at center stage and that takes the pressure off self-promotion. **You aren't promoting yourself, you're promoting transformation through yoga**, and that my friends, is worth promoting.

The purpose of every business is to serve its clients, but in order to do so, a business needs to get the word out about its existence. This is marketing: reaching out to people so they know you exist and you can actually help them. Sounds easy, right? The thing is there are a TON of businesses trying to grab people's attention and some of these businesses will sacrifice ethics in order to be heard. This is where mindful marketing comes into play. You don't have to be sneaky and manipulative in your marketing, but being heard amongst all the chatter takes strategy that is honest, smart and effective. I'll show you how.

Effective marketing is all about knowing your audience:

- What's important to them?
- What concerns them?

- Where and how do they spend their time?
- How can you serve them best?

It's also about knowing the ins-&-outs of what you offer. In refining a marketing plan with a teacher I recently coached, I asked what her marketing message was. She replied with, "I sell a peace of mind". That's a great start, at least she didn't say "I sell yoga", because by now you should recognize that we offer much more than merely yoga. A peace of mind answers the big picture question of what she offers, but it's not her all-encompassing message. So, I asked her again, "Yes, you sell a peace of mind, but what is the *message* behind it? Describe to me how you package that peace of mind to potential students". Her answer was simply a puzzled look.

This is not uncommon, as many teachers are confused about their marketing message. Some teachers think it's their slogan like CorePower Yoga's "Live Your Power", others think it's their vision or values, and some treat it as an overview of their accomplishments and teacher training certifications. It's actually none of these.

Although a slogan is definitely part of a marketing message, I want to be clear that it's not the whole enchilada. A well-crafted message grabs the prospect's attention, clearly portrays how you can help them, highlights your unique benefits, targets your particular audience, instills trust and always incorporates your branding. The key elements being attention grabbing and clearly communicating how you can make their life better.

CRAFTING YOUR MARKETING MESSAGE

Your marketing message should "speak" directly to your target audience. This is done by developing your message around thorough market research and using the precise language your audience used in your investigation and interviews. Remember the Market Research section? In addition to literature research and statistical data, I want you to get out there and talk directly with real people in your target audience (at least 5-10 of them). Find out exactly what their pain points are and what challenges they currently face that they would love a solution for. The words they use and the way they express their struggles are the meat-n-potatoes (or maybe you prefer tofu-n-potatoes) of being able to "speak" to your audience. Your marketing message is essentially the language you use on your website, the words you put on your flyers and the images you use on both. It's your way of communicating how you can help someone in a relatable manner.

Address these 6 components and ask yourself the following questions to create your successful marketing message:

1. **TARGET:** Does your messaging target your niche audience? As in, will the people you want to work with be able to relate to and hear your message? Or are you still trying to target everyone?

2. **ATTENTION:** Will it grab their attention? Are you addressing their pain points and challenges? Are you speaking their language? Can they see themselves in the images you use?

3. **TRANSFORMATION:** Do you clearly communicate how you will change their life for the better? How will you help them resolve their issues and overcome their obstacles?

4. **UNIQUENESS:** Have you highlighted your uniqueness in such a way that you stand out in the crowd? Is it obvious why they should choose you over the next teacher?

5. **TRUST:** Does it build trust and show you are trustworthy? Why should they believe you can help them? Here's a hint: because you've personally been in their shoes and/or you've helped someone else through it before. Testimonials, reviews, analytics and data are very helpful in building trust.

6. **BRAND:** Does your messaging align with your brand? Are you being consistent with it, from your website to social media posts to in-person conversations? Does your brand represent your message and does your message represent your brand?

Let's take a closer look at CorePower Yoga. If you aren't familiar with CorePower Yoga, they're known for plush studios with spa-like amenities, and set sequences that are exactly the same at every studio. Their studio model and branding might not resonate with you, but they execute their marketing strategy well, so hang in there, it's just an example. The CorePower message starts with "Live Your Power" and centers itself around the *experience* of practicing at their studios. In the CorePower experience, you will "Discover Your Most Powerful Self". On their website, the messaging continues with "Inside our yoga fitness studios, something amazing is happening. With this high intensity workout, you'll push past physical boundaries with an open mind and a beating heart, turning doubt into security, strangers into friends and stress into sweat".

Let's dissect that a bit further as it relates to our 6 components of successful messaging:

1. Do they target an audience? Yes, those looking for physical, asana yoga that's heavy on the workout, who enjoy feeling pampered, and value consistency in their experience.

2. Are they speaking their language? Absolutely, with words like "intensity", "workout", "power", "sweat" and "push".

3. Do they communicate a big picture of transformation? Yep, CorePower will help you discover your most powerful self through sweaty yoga that will open your mind, get your heart pumping, give you confidence, and release stress, all while making friends.

4. Do they point out what makes them unique? You bet ya. CorePower offers a variety of

"fitness yoga" classes, the studios are beautiful with spa-like amenities and the experience is consistent no matter the studio, city, or instructor.

5. Do they convey trust? Sort of. They use #whyiyoga to share people's experiences (which is a method displaying testimonials), but it's not very obvious in their messaging. The consistency of your experience in every studio could also be considered a form of trust, but overall, I think they could do better in this category.

6. Are they consistent with their branding? No doubt. From their name, slogan, color scheme, language and imagery, it all suggests "power", workout yoga, and creating change by pushing physical boundaries.

Marketing is all about being able to reach people and connect with them. When people are looking for someone to help them through a challenge, they want to know how you'll help them, which is different than what you do. **One of the biggest mistakes I see teachers make is focusing on What-I-Do instead of What-I-Can-Do-For-You.** That's why, in crafting your marketing message the most important component to focus on is TRANSFORMATION, aka What-I-Can-Do-For-You. In all of the ways that you share your business with people, focus on What-I-Can-Do-For-You, as opposed to What-I-Do.

Here's a classic example I see daily on Facebook that demonstrates how we can shift from What-I-Do to What-I-Can-Do-For-You. A teacher sharing her upcoming workshop in a post wrote:

"Feeling so blessed to be able to share this workshop. If you are interested in experiencing the healing journey through the lens of the chakras, join me for Chakra Healing & Kundalini Yoga on June 24. Price goes up in two weeks. Much love & Sat Nam."

First off, props for using social media as a means to promote and build your business, but let's be more effective with your approach. This post focuses almost entirely on What-I-Do, essentially saying here's my workshop, hope you'll come. If the goal is to motivate people to attend, What-I-Can-Do-For-You is much more motivating than What-I-Do.

Try something like this instead:

Ready for more balance and less stress? A healing journey awaits you on June 24th. Through the lens of the chakras, we'll travel inside to bust through your blocks and open your body and mind to the intuitive healing it needs. If you're ready to become the happiest and healthiest version of you, grab your spot now before the price goes up in 2 weeks. I can't wait to see your smiling face after this journey. Until then, much love and Sat Nam.

Now let's compare. The first post doesn't clearly explain what's in it for the attendee. The post infers to a healing journey, but the teacher doesn't specifically state the change she will help someone create. Plus, the overall tone doesn't exude confidence, nor does it have a strong call-to-action. The second post, however, obviously expresses what a person will gain from attending: less stress, balance, happiness, health and a smile. It doesn't just say "if you are interested in experiencing a healing journey," instead it announces that "a healing journey awaits you" which is much more confident and appealing. It also utilizes the question-first method of marketing. Posing a reflective question grabs the reader's attention and makes it personal. It helps the prospect get excited about what you're offering and serves as a segue into the greater message. Additionally, it builds in a call-to-action that's time sensitive and encourages people to act now and register.

PRO-TIP: When posing questions in our headlines and marketing messages, only use them when the answer is undoubtedly yes and segues into a greater message. Otherwise, the question you pose can work against your efforts.

CLIENT AVATAR

In creating your marketing plan, an avatar of your ideal client/student is really helpful. If you've been following along, then you've already done much of this work. It's basically all the market research you've done on you target audience, pulled together into an avatar-like profile. Said differently, it's an exercise to help you get really clear about the group you want to work with and is most likely to seek your service. Knowing your ideal client really well streamlines all of your marketing efforts because you know who you're speaking to, what they need and what motivates them to take action. Not only that, but you're more equipped to build out programs that truly create results for them.

WHAT AN IDEAL CLIENT IS:

- Someone who finds the perfect solution to their problems or needs in your service
- Someone who will personally connect with you and your brand, and is likely to refer you to their friends

WHAT AN IDEAL CLIENT IS NOT:

- A wish-list of you ideal BFF
- A perfect person

Contrary to some advice, don't focus your ideal client as being someone you would enjoy hanging out with. When we do that, we risk projecting our own ego and what we think they need into our client profile, instead of researching what their actual needs and characteristics are. When you paint the picture of your ideal client like a Stepford Wife, you sacrifice seeing them as a whole person, with struggles, challenges, and imperfections. Thus, they won't relate to your brand because they won't feel like you understand them.

A POOR AVATAR EXAMPLE

My ideal client is a busy mom who is health conscious, but needs help keeping up with her yoga practice, and has the income to pay for my services.

A BETTER AVATAR EXAMPLE

My ideal client is a busy mom working in the tech industry of the Silicon Valley. Prior to having kids, yoga was part of her active and healthy lifestyle, but these days, she struggles to find the time. When she factors in the time it takes to drive to the studio, find parking, and arrive early with the time of the class itself, it's unfeasible to her.

However, she's determined to find a solution. What she needs is a yoga teacher to come to her, saving her precious time that she can spend with her family. The convenience of at-home yoga is well worth the money, and she's got the budget for it. She knows that when she takes care of herself, she's better adept to care for her kids, so she's ready to commit to a regular practice.

As this is just a fictional example, your ideal client avatar will likely look completely different. What's essential though is identifying what motivates your ideal client. In the above scenario, the ideal client is motivated by her kids and being the best mom she can be. This is important to know so you can infuse that motivation into your marketing, ensuring your effectiveness and ability to attract the right kind of people.

Keep in mind: the profile of an ideal client should be based on observable characteristics, backed by data, research and actual conversations, not imagination or assumption.

ACTIVE & PASSIVE MARKETING

Ok, so now you have a client avatar and a marketing message to communicate what you offer. The next step is implementation. It's time to get out there and actually promote your business. Keep in mind, especially with face-to-face interactions, marketing isn't about promoting yourself, it's about promoting change and the benefits of yoga.

In marketing, there's two basic categories I want to discuss, passive and active marketing. Essentially, passive marketing helps prospects find you (think website, flyers and directories) while active marketing entails direct contact with prospects (think email, phone and in-person). It's no surprise that active marketing is one of the most underused approaches by yoga teachers. Why? Because the fear of rejection creeps back up. The thought of hearing a "no" face-to-face is just too frightening for some, and rightfully so. Rejection can be a debilitating feeling that may take hold in any stage of life. The thing to remember, though, is it's not about you. If you propose the idea of a private lesson to a colleague and they say "no thank you," recognize they're not really saying no to you. They're saying no to themselves and receiving the benefits of yoga. You can't take it personally. It might not be the right time in their life or maybe it never will be, but it's not about rejecting you.

Smart marketing combines both passive and active marketing. Balance direct interactions (face-to-face after a class) and indirect impressions (through your website or flyers) in a manner that works best for you.

Networking is a tremendously helpful form of active marketing. That means finding events and opportunities to meet and connect with people in your area and especially in your niche. For example, if you'd like to break into workplace/corporate yoga, check out your local chamber of commerce for all sorts of business events where you can meet people who own, manage and work at businesses in your area. The key to landing corporate gigs is having a direct inside referral, which often come from networking. The same goes for any niche, personal referrals and direct contacts will take you far, so get out there and start shaking some hands.

ONLINE PRESENCE

Being visible online is definitely part of your marketing plan. If you don't have a website, it's time to get one. However, your online presence can, and I suggest that it does, span beyond merely your website.

At minimum, your online marketing strategy should consist of these 3 components:

- A website
- An email list
- A social media channel

You see, **the key to marketing is being visible where people already spend time.** We've talked about this previously with two offline methods; partnering with businesses who already serve your niche audience and being at events they would attend such as conferences or networking meetings. Another approach is being visible where your target audience spends time online.

Example places and ways people spend time online are:

- Scrolling their social media feeds
- Reading articles and blog posts
- Chatting in discussion forums and Facebook groups

- Attending online summits and conferences
- Reading and responding to emails
- Shopping for products and services
- Watching videos on YouTube

Let's say your work is centered around techies and you help them counterbalance the side effects of working at a computer all day.

Here's a few ways you can make your services visible to techies online:

1. Engage with individuals on social media as well as prominent tech figures and businesses who could give you exposure
2. Publish an article in a tech publication about the benefits of yoga for techies and link to your website in the article itself and/or in your bio at the end of the article
3. Similar to the previous suggestion, guest-post on a tech-blog and link back to your website
4. Provide value to people by contributing to discussions on tech forums and link to your services when it's appropriate
5. As you grow your audience with an email list, continue nurturing those relationships with

email broadcasts that provide helpful information as well as promote your services
6. Expose your business to techies by creating free video classes on YouTube that promote your brand and drive traffic to your website
7. Advertise your services on tech websites or blogs

Content Marketing

People have become immune to traditional methods of marketing, myself included. We DVR our favorite shows and fast-forward through the commercials, we swiftly skip over magazine ads, and we're quick to spot a sponsored post in our feed and ignore it. We don't trust a company through a simple advertisement anymore. We search out more information on their website, we get to know the business, we read reviews and we take note of their reputation overtime. People are simply tired of being "sold" to all the time, especially when we didn't seek out the business or service to begin with.

So, how would you feel if I told you there's another approach to marketing that doesn't involve in-your-face selling? If that excites you, then let me introduce to you to *content marketing*, your new best friend! In the expert words of the Content Marketing Institute, "Content marketing is a strategic marketing approach focused on creating and distributing valuable, relevant, and consistent content to attract and retain a clearly defined audience - and, ultimately, to drive profitable customer action."

To really understand content marketing, let's start by looking at what content is. A blog post, an infographic, a video, and an eBook are all forms of content. Content is both information and communication. Through a video, we can communicate an idea or message and share valuable information. Thus, the idea behind content marketing is sharing useful information as a means of communicating to prospects, without hard-selling.

With so much information available at our fingertips and almost every business, service or product having some type of searchable existence online, we prefer to seek out what we need, when we need it. As opposed to having advertisements in our face all the time. So, you can think of content marketing as a method that works when people need to find you. It's like planting seeds around on the internet that all lead back to you. For example, if you've published a few targeted articles, partnered with a few niche businesses who've linked back to you, and made yourself accessible on numerous directories (both yoga and niche related) then you've strategically placed breadcrumbs around that will all help people find you when they Google your niche keywords.

Blogging is a great example to show how content marketing is applicable. Have you ever gone to a restaurant's website and wondered why they have a blog? It's more than likely, the restaurant is using the blog as a means of content marketing. By providing helpful information around food and cooking, their blog generates exposure around their business and traffic to their website.

Refer back to our techie example in the previous section. **Building your online presence can be interchangeable with content marketing.** For instance, guest-posting on a tech blog simultaneously builds your online presence while communicating to prospects that you are there to help them. Here's how.

The readers of a tech blog are primarily techies, so you've got your target audience. First, get to know the blog by observing the blogger's writing style and what type of posts get the most engagement. Based on that, come up with a post that will suit the blog and the audience. Your post could be something like this - Yoga Hacks: How To Undue The Stress Of Spending So Much Time At Your Computer. 99% of your focus should be on providing highly useful, highly relevant information. Use the other 1% to insert a correlation to your business. Some bloggers will allow you to speak directly about your service in the body of the content itself, but most prefer you leave it for your bio. Every blog post or article you submit to a publication will provide a section for you to include an author bio. Make the most of your bio by relating it to the post content and linking to your most relevant website page.

With this type of approach to marketing, you're accomplishing a few things at once:

- Establishing your expertise
- Providing valuable information that helps people
- Connecting with a target audience in a meaningful way
- Exposing your brand to a target audience

- Creating a backlink to your website that will improve your SEO (aka Google ranking)
- Growing your audience and email list
- Building a relationship with a recognized expert and potential business partner

However, traditional marketing methods are still helpful and aren't obsolete. The marketing landscape is just shifting and changing, but all the basic elements are still there. A marketing plan optimized for your highest success will include active, passive, traditional and content marketing.

Social Media

When it comes to social media, the first thing to know is that **you don't have to be everywhere**. Teachers get very overwhelmed by the idea of not only establishing a website, but a Facebook page, Twitter handle, Pinterest board, YouTube channel, Instagram account etc. Phew, that's a lot of places to be and is understandably overwhelming. Nevertheless, you don't have to stand on every platform, but I highly suggest at least one.

Social media gets a bad rap sometimes, and for many valid reasons, but when you acknowledge what it's done for the world, it's hard to ignore its beneficial impact. Social media has changed the way we respond to natural disasters, has united voices around the globe highlighting international injustices, and has given us access to real-time accounts of events unfiltered by the news media. All the while it helps non-profits raise money, keeps us connected with friends, and gives us a place to post selfies. It has its good and its bad, but at the core of it all, **social media is all about relationships and connecting people**.

What does this mean for you and your business?

1. **Build & Nurture Relationships:** Social media isn't about hard-selling. It's about getting to know one another, and sharing your message. It's a place to interact with both prospects and current clients, and nurture those relationships. On social media, people can find you and you can find them without the hard-sell.

2. **Motivate & Inspire:** Because people use social media on a daily basis it's a great platform to provide some daily love and inspiration to your audience. Whether it's a

case study, a motivational message, or an informative article, you can enrich people's lives with a daily connection to your teachings.

3. **<u>Global Voice:</u>** Social media has given small businesses a global voice. The reach that once cost a business thousands of dollars, can now be achieved virtually for free. However small you think your niche may be, expand your reach across oceans and watch it grow beyond what you ever imagined.

4. **<u>Client Insight:</u>** Among all the photos, videos and comments is a wealth of information about your target audience - what they like, what they don't, how they react, and how they feel about you. Pay mindful attention and you'll learn a great deal.

A WORD ABOUT FACEBOOK & INSTAGRAM

Facebook is great for its ability to share mixed media, i.e. photos, videos, articles, memes, events and more. I also like Facebook for its business features such as the "book now" call-to-action button. However, Facebook's biggest downside for a business is their use of an algorithm to display posts instead of using chronological order. Because so many people and businesses are posting on Facebook, a very large percentage of posts are never seen by users when they're shown in a feed with real-time. Thus, Facebook has developed an algorithm to show a user 300 of the most relevant posts each time they sign on. This way, Facebook reduces the likelihood that you miss an important (relevant) post just because you logged on 3 hours after it was posted.

This algorithm has evolved over the years from favoring high-quality content to downgrading text-only posts to paid for boosts, and it will only continue to evolve. But know this, businesses are at a disadvantage. Even though your followers have "liked" your page because they want to read your posts, your organic reach can be minuscule. Businesses are outraged by the fact that out of 2,000 follows, their post only reaches 200 of them because of this algorithm. Don't be fooled by Instagram or Twitter either. Although implemented much more recently, they both use similar algorithms to decide what you see in your feed. So, what's my point?

Don't put all your marketing eggs into the social media basket. Yes, there's undeniable potential for growth and connection with social media, however, be cautious with how you spend your time, energy and money. Why? Because email may turn out to be your more prominent means of communicating. While it becomes increasingly harder for a business to engage with its followers on social media, a person's email inbox remains in their complete control - no algorithm that decides what shows up.

EMAIL LIST

Social media is great for outreach, but the next step is transitioning followers to your email list - the central hub of your communication network. In fact, many experts say your email list is the single most important asset to your business, and I agree.

For most independent yoga teachers, email is the most effective means of communicating with your audience because:

- Email is still the most used form of online communication

- You have a direct line of communication that isn't subject to Facebook or anyone else's decisions. You own your list.
- Your subscribers opted-in which shows a stronger interest and commitment level then hitting a "like" button

Again, like content marketing and social media, your email list is about relationships and providing value, not hard-selling. The key to successful email marking is finding a balance between providing useful content and relevant information about your business. Research shows it takes 5-10 impressions or interactions before a person decides to book with you or purchase something. Thus, the more relevant and valuable your emails are, the more trust and credibility you earn with them - and the more likely they are to work with you when they're ready.

Here are examples of content pieces to include in your emails (aka, newsletter, broadcast or campaign):

- Words of inspiration (quotes, passages from the Yoga Sutras, your own words of advice, etc.)

- Motivational messages (reminders to practice and to practice with *you*)
- A short blurb and link to your recent, value-packed blog post
- A link to an outside informative/helpful article
- Ayurveda tips for balanced eating
- Healthy lifestyle tips
- Your public class schedule (and any changes being made to it)
- Upcoming workshops, retreats and other events
- Special offers and discounts
- Information on your latest online course or eBook
- A link to the free online class you just published on YouTube
- Your latest meditation download

Don't forget, people voluntarily sign-up for your email list because they want to hear from you. It's not spam. Plus, they can opt-out anytime they want, so don't be afraid to communicate. Another helpful tip is frontloading your value-based content. That is, put the motivational message and lifestyle tips first, then follow it up with your schedule and other offerings. Doing so serves a dual purpose: by providing some sort of value first then inviting them to join your workshop feels much less promotional, and it keeps your non-local audience interested, as they don't have to scroll through your local schedule to find your meditation video.

Most importantly, start building your list now! Even if you aren't ready to start utilizing your list, don't wait to collect email addresses until you have something to say. Collect emails now from anyone who resonates with you, and you'll have a list when you're ready. For teachers and entrepreneurs who've come to use their email lists successfully, their only regret is that they wish they started sooner. **With proper use and a little time to grow, your email list will no doubt help fill your classes, sell-out your workshops, and transition prospects to booked clients.**

How to Get Subscribers

Now that you know *why* you need an email list, let's talk about *how* you get folks to subscribe.

I can clearly recall the first time I heard a teacher share their email list with a public studio class. That teacher was Charanpal Kaur, remember her from the retreat section? Sitting in bliss moments after her class came to a close, I observed students quickly approaching her with comments and questions. As others began to roll up their mats, Charanpal paused and announced to the group that she sends out helpful advice and updates on her teachings through her newsletter. As she pulled out her clipboard, students began to jot down their emails with the same enthusiasm they displayed as they approached her with questions. Feeling so much happiness from my experience in Charanpal's class, I too eagerly signed-up to her newsletter to get as much Charanpal in my life as I could.

What I want to point out is how easy it was and how she leveraged the valuable moments after class. People related to Charanpal and felt moved by the teachings she shared, so it was an effortless decision to want to stay connected with her. No one felt solicited, because we saw so much value in what she was offering, and you can do the same.

First of all, whenever you're teaching in-person, bring your sign-up clipboard. Put it in your yoga bag along with your journal, canteen and other items you may carry with you to classes, so it's always there to use. Charanpal suggests, "If you deliver a good experience, they feel really good, and they want more, that's the time" - after classes and workshops, and at events. She emphasizes the strength of a connection made in-person.

Second, don't be afraid to invite people to join. A simple mention is all it takes. Charanpal explains, "Those who sign-up are curious enough and if they end up unsubscribing (which doesn't happen often) you can't take it personally. It just means they're not as interested. And the truth is, you really want to have people on that list who are interested".

Third, put your website to work for you. Every visitor who comes to your site should be invited to join. Maybe they aren't ready to book a private session right away, but if they're curious enough and willing to take a small step, they'll sign-up for your email list. It's a great sign of potential and shows they're interested in what you offer. This way, you can continue to provide them value, and when the time is right, they'll more than likely choose you as the teacher they decide to work with.

OFFER A FREE GIFT

A really fun way to build your email list is by incentivizing people with a free gift in return for signing up. Generally speaking, this gift should be in digital form. Something that doesn't cost you anything to create except a bit of time, and can be automatically delivered to the subscriber through your email list auto-responder. When you set up your email list sign-up form through your email marketing provider, you'll be prompted to create a welcome or thank you email that will automatically be sent after someone subscribes. This is where you'll include a link (or button) for your subscriber to download your gift. By the way, you'll want to upload the gift itself to your website beforehand and use that link in your welcome message as a means to access the gift. Don't worry if you're confused by this process a bit. Your email provider will probably have a tutorial and if for some reason they don't, you can find one through a Google search.

Be creative when coming up with your free gift and explore your entire skill set, but be sure it's something that will appeal to your niche. The more helpful and valuable it is, the more people will trust you and look forward to your emails.

Some examples are:

- Your ultimate guide to healthy living
- An audio download of a guided meditation to release stress
- A 20-minute yoga video to ease low-back pain
- A dosha quiz to determine one's Ayurvedic constitution
- A beautiful PDF of your favorite green smoothie recipes

Email Service Provider

Lastly, you'll need a service provider to create and deliver your newsletter with. Mailchimp is free for your first 1,000 subscribers and is really easy to use (www.mailchimp.com). They have pre-designed, yet customizable templates and sign-up forms that you can easily embed into your website. Of course, the free option doesn't come with all the bells and whistles, so you'll miss out on a few things automation. Aweber is another great provider I highly recommend and they boast very similar features to Mailchimp (www.aweber.com). Aweber's free option is a 30-day trail, and they don't restrict you from automation.

When I say automation, what I'm referring to is the ability to use an auto-responder, which allows you send a message or sequence of messages automatically to your subscribers. For example, if you want to send your free gift or a thank you email with special offers after someone subscribes, you'll want to use an auto-responder. Instead of having to manually send your gift to each subscriber, your auto-responder will send it immediately after they subscribe.

You may also want to include some follow up emails that will also be automatically delivered. For example, a few days after your gift has been delivered you may want to ask your subscriber how they liked it and if they have any questions. For a third email in the sequence, perhaps you'll want to send another similar offer that would interest them. Or maybe you want your free gift or a product you offer to be delivered over a specific time period. For instance, your ultimate guide to healthy living can be presented as a 4-week course, program or challenge that's broken down into four weekly emails, each containing a different lesson and component of your guide. You'll need to set this email sequence up with your auto-responder.

For the auto-responder feature, you'll need to pay for Mailchimp or use Aweber.

WEBSITE

As I said before, a website is a must for any business, which means it's time for you to not only create a website, but actually utilize it to help your business grow. Think of your website like your business listing back in the good ol' days of the Yellow Pages. Whether you're finding a new studio, researching a product you wish to buy, or looking for an old friend, the first place people go is the internet. The same is true for yoga instruction. These days, flyers and personal referrals will only take potential clients so far along the path to booking. After coming in contact with your flyer, a prospect's next step would be to look up your website to find more information. In this regard, a strong website has the power to convert a potential client into a booked client, whether it's a corporate gig, a private Skype session or a retreat. You are a business and in this day and age, every business should have a website.

Your website is your personal corner of the internet to build your community and attract clients 24/7. It's a place where people can:

- Find you
- Get to know you
- Learn about your services and their benefits
- Contact you
- Purchase and book private sessions
- Sign-up for your email list
- Register for workshops
- Take your online classes and more

Building & Hosting

Rest assured, websites are cheap and easy to create nowadays. A simple Google search will reveal loads of options to develop and host your site without needing to hire an expensive web designer.

If you aren't familiar with the way websites work, there are three basic components:

1. **Domain:** your web address (the website name)
2. **Building:** putting together your site page by page (the content itself)
3. **Hosting:** a place to store your website (essentially the server where it lives)

When deciding on a service provider it's helpful to know what you're looking for. Some companies are hosting providers, some are builders and some are both. You'll also need to register your domain name, which will be done through whatever company supports your hosting.

Here are three recommendations in order of what I consider beginner, intermediate and advanced:

1. **Weebly** (www.weebly.com): If you don't know where to start and often find yourself saying "I'm not very tech-savvy" I highly recommend Weebly because it's an all-in-one platform. With Weebly you can register your domain name, build your site and host it all with the same provider. The design

process is simple, it's very user-friendly and it's cheap. Weebly is perfect for the newbie, but naturally a bit limiting for someone who wants more customization and special features.

2. **Squarespace** (www.squarespace.com): Very much like Weebly in that it's a one-stop-shop platform and comes equipped with lots of design templates. Squarespace has a few more customization options and cool features than Weebly, which is great, but that comes with a slightly higher learning curve. The designs are also optimized for visuals and imagery, which could be positive or negative depending on what your business needs and your preferences are. In terms of price, the basic packages are only a couple of bucks more than Weebly.

3. **Wordpress** (www.wordpress.org): My suggestion if you want full customization, intricate tools and all the bells and whistles. There are paid design themes, but they also have free options. However, Wordpress is just a builder, so you'll still need a hosting provider, such as BlueHost (www.bluehost.com), which adds to the complexity of your site setup, but is still

feasible. If statistics tell you anything, 74.6 million sites are supported by Wordpress, and for good reason. For robust functionality, customization and integration, Wordpress just can't be beat. That said, the learning curve is definitely higher, but well worth it when you're ready.

In conclusion, if you've never built a website before, try Weebly or Squarespace. If you've got some experience or you already know Weebly and Squarespace don't offer features you need, then go with Wordpress. Additionally, all three platforms have plenty of free tutorials on the internet, so try not to get frustrated learning the platform. If you get stuck, just Google a few keywords and you'll likely find a written or video tutorial to help you out.

Quality Content

Now, before you get all tied up in color schemes and photos, the most critical component of your site is content. **Without quality content that serves a purpose, your website can easily become cluttered with junk and gibberish.** Remember, your website (like your other marketing tools) should center around What-I-Can-Do-For-You, not What-I-Do. Don't overload your website with photos of you in complex asanas and an extensive bio on the front page. If a visitor doesn't see the value in your website within seconds (yes, only seconds) they'll hit the back button and return to their search. Thus, you need to let a visitor know right away what you can do for them. Sure, people want to know who you are, but that's what the *about me* page is for. Not your *home* page.

Each page on your site should have one specific goal or intention, and designed to point visitors in that direction. In the case of your *home* page, you need to grab their attention and entice them to stay on your site and explore it further. This is another place where having a niche and conducting solid market research comes in handy. Without a niche and a message that resonates with that unique group, you'll lose a ton of visitors to the back button because it's not clear from the get-go that you can help them.

Thus, the intention behind your *home* page is to catch the visitor's attention with your marketing message and direct the them to the next step. Depending on your business model, this next step might be to book a private session, view your latest online class or read your recent blog post. However, for most of us, the next step will be to sign-up for your email list. Once they're on your email list, even if the hit the back button right after, you have the ability to be in contact with them and continue providing value until they're ready to work with you. By the way, not every visitor will land on your *home* page first. Some might come to your site via a blog page, so it's important to have multiple email sign-up forms throughout your website.

Keep this idea of intention in mind while building out your website. What specific goal will each page have? What's the purpose of the page and what action do you want visitors to take? This is will not only help visitors navigate your website, but will give you clarity in building it out. As the website developer, we often forget that visitors are in a hurry and the harder we make it for them to find the info they're looking for, the quicker they'll leave. The key element, and sometimes the hardest to achieve, is simplicity - less is more.

Here are a few points to consider that can overhaul simplicity:

- Too much text (irrelevant/non-essential information)
- Poor placement of essential information (vital info should be bolded, front-loaded and clearly visible by scanning)
- Not enough repetition (your messaging should be consistent on each page, and make good use of keywords)
- Improper use of calls-to-action (just as not having a call-to-action will lead to inactivity, so can too many options)
- Too many photos (images help to convey a message, but too many will distract from your message)

BRANDING

Marketing and branding are like yin and yang - interconnected yet separate forces. Branding should precede and underlie any marketing efforts. While marketing is more about demonstrating the value of what you offer, branding is an expressive representation of your business values and attributes as a whole. Marketing is a tactical approach to being heard and seen, while branding is what's left after your marketing message does its job. Your marketing efforts may convince someone to work with you, but your brand is what keeps them coming back. A brand is what people remember and recommend to their friends.

Said beautifully by John Williams in Entrepreneur, "Defining your brand is like a journey of business self-discovery. It can be difficult, time-consuming and uncomfortable" (www.entrepreneur.com/article/77408).

He continues, "It requires, at the very least, that you answer the questions below:

- What is your company's mission?
- What are the benefits and features of your products or services?
- What do your customers and prospects already think of your company?
- What qualities do you want them to associate with your company?"

Answering these questions all comes down to clarity around what you offer and how you can visually express it. What images or symbols signify your message, what words convey your values, what colors represent the transformation you provide? Visually expressive, how can you tie everything together in a meaningful, aesthetically pleasing and consistent representation of your business?

Don't sweat it if you can't clearly see your brand yet. Branding takes time and even changes as a business grows. If you're just starting out, don't get hung-up on branding to a point where it postpones getting your business up and running. Especially if you're still working out your niche. However, if you find it comes relatively easy, branding from the beginning can be very helpful in building your business.

Lifestyle guru and yoga teacher Yely Staley (aforementioned in the tour section), is an inspiring example of a teacher who began the process of branding early on (www.yogayely.com). Before she even completed teacher training, Yely had a clear vision of how she wanted to portray herself to the community and let her personality shine. Part of that was sharing the transition from student to teacher and being truly authentic in communicating her journey. As humans, we all change and grow, and Yely knew people could identify with that, so she let it come forth as part of her brand.

For Yely, her brand is an expression of her professionalism and commitment to her career as a teacher. It was very important for her to present herself as an enthusiastic and reliable professional with a vision, and her brand brings that together. Even though her brand will shift and grow, sharing her intimate evolution is very much part of the Yoga Yely brand.

In developing your brand consider these tips:

1. Get personal. People relate to other humans, so share your personality and have fun with it.
2. Be unique. What's your niche? Why you? What's different about your brand?
3. Grow your community. Like we talked about with content marketing, **build relationships and trust in your brand by being a valuable contributor to your niche community.**
4. Deliver outstanding service. No matter where you're at in your career and

experience teaching, do your absolute best and people will notice.

5. Be consistent. In your colors, images and messaging, consistency is important to expressing your values and building brand recognition.

CHAPTER 7:
KNOW YOUR VALUE

It's one thing to offer your services for free in order to gain experience and/or refine a program, but it's an entirely different thing to not understand your worth. This is a very common struggle for teachers, but can be resolved with awareness and action. If you find yourself thinking, "It's not spiritual to charge for my work", "I'm not worthy of earning abundantly" or "I'm not good enough to charge this much" then it's time to work through your blocks.

SHIFT YOUR MONEY MINDSET

The first step to financial abundance is recognizing that you have a gift to share with the world. A gift that's extremely valuable, as it heals and transforms both individuals and societies. **If you aren't able to earn from this gift, then you won't be able to share it in the same capacity you could otherwise.**

Remember, you have to put on your oxygen mask before helping others. Earning from your work enables you to serve more and give more, so let your work support you. Accept it and own it. Say a mantra and meditate on owning your earning potential until your fear dissolves. It's spiritually OK to earn, it's simply an exchange of energy.

The second step is feeling out your earning potential. Pricing is a process that often changes with experience and time, so take your time with it. Don't charge something just because it's what everyone else is charging. You have to feel out your work and come to understand its worth through experience. If you're insecure about your work as a whole and why you charge what you do, fear will arise when you discuss pricing and people will be able to sense your insecurity. It circles back to the first step of understanding the value in the work you do. That's what generates confidence in your pricing and financial abundance.

Step three is identifying your blocks. What's your personal story about your earning potential? What blocks your creative earning capacity? Write it down in compete honesty in your journal. Then take a look at your language and begin the process of changing your patterns. Transform "I'm not worthy" to "The world needs my work and I am worthy of receiving in exchange". Shift your energy from a place of fear and lack to a place of confidence and prosperity.

AVOID DROP-INS

When it comes to pricing, I encourage you to steer clear of offering your services on a drop-in basis. Whether you rent space from a studio or other facility, you teach a weekly class in the park or you teach a corporate class in which the employees pay themselves, try to come up with a different framework for your pricing, such as a prepaid class series or monthly rate.

Looking at traditional studios, the drop-in model doesn't lend itself to consistency for the student's practice, the teacher's salary or the studio's revenue. When different folks are continuously revolving in and out of classes, the drop-in model doesn't make for a strong community environment either. Now I'm not saying that drop-in studios aren't successful, clearly many of them are, but the drop-in model is not the most conducive to commitment and regularity.

Gyms are a great example of an alternative model that studios are picking up. They require monthly memberships, which in turn, produces much more consistency across the board. In generating your pricing structure, consider what makes the most sense for your business and optimizes your pricing system. While monthly memberships are awesome, they might not be suitable to your business model, so let's discuss another option - packages.

PACKAGES CREATE CONSISTENCY

Another part about pricing teachers commonly overlook is how their pricing structure impacts their schedule, consistency, commitment and the perceived value of their service. Whatever your niche, whether you teach corporate classes or private Skype sessions, work towards consistency and long-term clients.

Let's start this discussion by looking at the common approach to packaging for private classes that involves an incentive to buy more, and looks something like this:

- Single (1 hour) session $95
- Pack of 3 (1 hour) sessions $255 ($85 each)
- Pack of 6 (1 hour) sessions $450 ($75 each)

What's great about this tiered structure is that it creates an incentive for clients to buy bulk classes upfront with a decrease in price. Purchasing upfront packages shows commitment, as they are ready to invest in you, their practice, and their health. A client who buys a single session at a time isn't ready to commit, which is generally why they won't buy a package (even with the savings they'll receive). Maybe they aren't sure if they'll be able to find the time and money or perhaps they're still unsure if it'll be worth their while, and often they just generally lack the motivation to take action on their desires.

Packages equal commitment and consistency. Students who are committed or willing to commit are the best type of clients for your yoga business. Whether students are committing to a package, a long-term contract (think corporate gigs) or a class series, it all equates to consistency in their practice and time with you. This in turn creates consistency not only in their progress, but in your schedule and income. With your clients purchasing packages and booking ahead, you know what to expect in your schedule week to week. Knowing your schedule in advance allows you to plan your weeks and book new students with confidence. With that kind of regularity, you also know what to expect from your income month to month. With more consistency in your schedule and income, the easier it becomes to create your ideal schedule, optimize your time, make accurate financial projections, and achieve your business goals.

The next question becomes; do you even offer a single session, be it privates, corporate or coaching calls? Some yoga teachers don't offer a single session as a way to weed out the non-committers. To them, it's a matter of time, suitability, and business goals. Their ideal client is ready to commit, so they don't want to waste time filling their schedules with one-timers who won't be there the following week.

It's up to you, however, and depends on how you want to operate your business and reach your goals. The benefit to offering a single session is that sometimes people just need to take you for a test run. A single session can act as a trial session to see if student and teacher are suitable for one another. This can be especially true for beginners and corporate teaching. If you decide to offer single sessions, consider offering it as in **introductory, one-time only session**. That is, a client can only buy a single session once. After the first introduction class, they can only purchase packages.

If your business model is based more on virtual teaching, aiming for consistency and long-term clients still applies. You could sell "one-off" classes, but it'd be more lucrative and helpful for your students to commit to a package of classes or services. Better yet, a monthly membership option lends to even more regularity in your income and client results.

Value Packages

There's another type of package you can create within your pricing structure that I like to call value packaging. This type of package is all about creating more value for your student, not just more sessions.

Think about going to your local car wash. The pricing structure builds more value into each tier and looks something like this:

- Basic Wash: $12 (includes: exterior wash and window cleaning)
- Full Service: $24 (includes: exterior wash, window cleaning, interior vacuum, and wax)
- The Works: $36 (includes: exterior wash, window cleaning, interior vacuum, wax, tire cleaning, underbody flush, and air freshener)

With value packages, each pricing tier offers more value through additional services or support.

For yoga teachers, the added value usually comes in the form of:

- Longer sessions
- Support emails
- Phone check-ins
- Yoga equipment (mats, blocks, etc.)
- Video/audio class downloads
- Meditation downloads

- Tailored sequences for the student's home practice (can include printouts with asana descriptions)
- Physical assessments and goal assessments
- Additional specialties & modalities (massage, nutrition consulting, Reiki, etc.)
- PDF guides
- Access to a private Facebook group
- Admission to webinars
- One-on-one coaching calls
- An eBook

I'll give you an example:

Justin is a private yoga teacher who is also a certified nutrition coach. He's blended his passions and created this value-based pricing structure for his clients:

1. **Beginner Yogi** (3-week series): Physical assessment, nutrition assessment, 6 private yoga sessions (60 minutes each), and Gaiam Eco Mat. $450.
2. **Inspired Yogi** (4-week series): Physical assessment, nutrition assessment, 8 private yoga sessions (75 minutes each), 4-week meal plan, 2 at-home sequences, 4 check-in

phone calls and Gaiam Eco Mat and block. $750.

3. **Avid Yogi** (5-week series): Physical assessment, nutrition assessment, 10 private yoga sessions (90 minutes each), 5-week meal plan, 3 at-home sequences, 3 audio meditation downloads, 5 check-in phone calls and Gaiam Eco mat, block and strap. $1,050.

This would also apply to online courses and themed programs. Let's say you have an online prenatal course. Instead of just one option that packs in your complete course, you could create three different options. Starting with the lowest price point, each tier would offer more value at a slightly higher price. This way people can find one that fits their budget. A little hint, most will opt for your middle option.

A WORD ON DISCOUNTS

Working discounts into your pricing structure is a controversial topic. Numerous marketing professionals say discounts are an effective strategy to get more clients. However, there are just as many experts claiming discounts devalue your service and diminish loyalty. In my experience, I've found discounts work in certain circumstances, but can be a hindrance in others. It really depends on your teaching experience, niche, client base, and business goals.

I've seen many new teachers (myself included) get their first private clients by offering discounts to their close community (friends, fellow yogis, colleagues, family, etc.). When people know you personally, they know the discount isn't a reflection of desperation or poor quality. However, those could be the exact qualities a discount portrays to those who don't know you. While discounts can be a great way to gain experience, test new waters, and sway potential clients on the fence, those clients are not likely to stick around.

When deciding whether or not to offer discounts, consider the following points:

- It's very likely they aren't ready to commit. Someone who isn't willing to make a full price financial investment probably isn't ready to commit to being a long-term client with you. That's not good for consistency and predictability with your business goals.

- They'll expect more discounts. If a client comes in at a low price, they'll often expect that price to continue (surprisingly even when they know it was a one-time offer). They'll wait for your next sale/discount, or they'll move onto the next yoga teacher offering cheap classes (think of Groupon addicts).

- It sets the tone for your service. If you follow up a discounted $25 session with a $75 session where nothing has changed except the sequence (i.e. no more value has been added to your service), you may find your clients confused about why the full price is so much higher when you've already set the tone for a $25 value

CHAPTER 8:
POLICIES & LEGAL
MATTERS

POLICIES

Whether your business features private sessions, one-on-one coaching, teacher trainings or a virtual yoga studio, you'll want to develop policies that establish expectations and protect you in certain circumstances. A policy is a statement of intent or system of principals to guide decisions. You'll likely run into a number of situations where it's helpful to have such a system in place. Policies inform your client of what outcomes they can expect in certain situations, and outline a protocol for you to follow in the instance of say, a last-minute cancellation.

Generally, policies take time and experience to develop as situations unique to your niche reveal themselves. For example, if your niche involves children, you may need a policy regarding age requirements. Or if you travel to the homes of your clients, you may want to establish a service area and include a travel fee for those outside that area. Although this takes time, it's important to think about boundaries and set up a few foundational policies. Once you have your policies established, bring them together into one document and have each client sign it before you begin your work together. The following are examples of common policies you'll likely need to establish.

Cancellations

A cancellation policy is probably one of the most important policies you'll need to write because they happen often. Life doesn't always go as planned, nor do our days and sometimes people need to cancel. I've had corporate clients cancel, coaching calls cancel and missed classes in a group series. Therefore, it's necessary to think about how you will handle such a situation ahead of time.

Most commonly, teachers set forth a 24-hour cancellation policy. That is, a client must contact you at least 24 hours prior to the scheduled time. When enforcing such a policy, it's imperative to consider what your time is worth. With proper notice, could you have scheduled someone else or done something productive with that time? What happens if someone cancels while you are on your way there or via an email that you haven't checked yet?

Often, these are tricky situations to deal with, but a clearly stated policy will help. Consider what your time is worth and how you'd like to handle cancellations. Decide if you will change a client full price, half price or anything at all if they don't provide you with 24-hours notice. Additionally, consider what will happen if you need to cancel. What will your protocol be in that situation?

Tardiness

A tardy policy directly relates to what your time is worth as well. If a client is 10 minutes late for a session, is it your duty to stay 10 minutes past your scheduled time? And what if you're late? What will your plan be to handle the situation? Think it through and write it out.

Missed Classes

When conducting a group class series, you'll definitely want a policy to address missed classes. Decide what you want to do in the circumstance that a registered student has to miss a class or two within your series. If the student knows ahead of time that they'll be out of town, some teachers prefer to handle it by giving them a discount on the total price. Other teachers record (either audio or video) each class, so anyone who misses one can take the class at home. Yet others offer makeup classes outside the scheduled classes. Be careful with that option, though, because you have to think about what your time is worth. Especially if your group is small or you only have one series going at a time, makeup classes can end up costing you more than they are worth.

Payments

Payment policies can be complicated depending on the options you offer for collecting payments. To ensure simplicity, streamline your accepted payment methods and establish clear boundaries about when payment is expected. When using electronic methods of payment, don't over-complicate things by accepting PayPal, Stripe, and Square. Instead, choose one. Based on your preference, establish one option for when payment is due. For example, either require pre-payment for everyone or invoice your clients weekly or monthly. Additionally, think about how you will handle refunds and include a refund policy.

Expiration Dates

Be sure to include expiration dates on packages. Otherwise, they can be drawn out over months, even years. You'll have to decide for yourself based on the unique qualities of your niche and how you want to operate. Generally, I give expiration dates that are 30% - 50% longer in time than the indented time of use. So, for a six session package designed for three weeks (two classes per week), I would give the sessions a four or five week expiration date. Example wording: When purchasing a package, all six sessions must be used within five weeks of the purchase date.

Remember the rules about consistency. You know you won't be delivering the same results if your client drags out their sessions (or whatever it is your package offers) over months due to your lenient expiration dates. Expiration dates help keep them on track and your schedule predictable.

Payment Plans

People can't always pay for packages or expensive courses upfront, so offering payment plans can be a huge benefit. On the other hand, payment plans can be risky if they aren't implemented with proper precaution.

Do not let payment plans extend beyond the time you and your client are working together. For example, if they purchased a three-week package, do not let the installments span over four weeks. It can get confusing if they continue to purchase packages. Additionally, make sure they sign an agreement to your payment plan so they are held accountable and don't bail on you half way through. PayPal even has a feature to let you set up recurring payments directly through your website, as do most of the other

payment service providers
(https://www.paypal.com/us/webapps/mpp/pro-
recurring-payments).

LEGAL MATTERS

Liability Waiver

A Waiver of Liability, sometimes called a Release of
Liability, is a legal form that acknowledges the risks
involved with yoga and attempts to remove you, the
business, from liability in an incident of injury. You
should have each and every student you teach sign
your waiver form before you begin to work together,
including all in-person sessions and Skype sessions.

Enforceability of such a form depends on state law,
a jury and the language of the waiver, thus it's highly
recommended that you consult with a local attorney
to draft your waiver around your local regulation. If
you cannot afford to pay an attorney, seek out your
local SBA (Small Business Association) and find out

if your city has a community program that offers free or low cost legal counseling. You can also find a fair amount of legal advice and sample documents online with a simple Google search. Additionally, yoga teacher and attorney, Gary Kissiah, has written many books on legal matters concerning the yoga business (www.garykissiah.com).

Keep in mind, liability for negligent and reckless teaching can never be waived. Your best protection is to:

- Continuously educate yourself about risks, injuries and the biomechanics of yoga
- Use careful teaching practices
- Be honest with your students if you don't know how to reasonably care for a special condition
- Arm yourself with sufficient liability insurance

Liability Insurance

It's unfortunate that we have to worry about lawsuits, but it's important to understand that as a result of being an independent contractor, we are sole proprietors. This means you are the business entity and personally liable. Thus, your personal assets are the business assets and your home, car and other such valuable properties can be taken as part of a legal award.

Insurance is crucial for any yoga teacher. Even if you teach at a studio, liability is likely shared. Sufficient insurance will help protect you from paying out of pocket for damage claims in the event of a lawsuit. Take it from Gary Kissiah, in a Yoga Alliance article from 2014 he writes, "Yoga, a $7 billion industry in the United States, continues to grow each year and, consequently, so do the legal risks associated with teaching the practice or running a studio" (https://www.yogaalliance.org/Learn/Legal_Essentials_for_Yoga_Teachers_and_Studios).

A quality insurance policy will cover most styles of yoga and some bodywork. However, when choosing a policy, in the same article Gary suggests, "One the most important sections of any policy describes what is excluded from coverage by the policy. For example, acroyoga, aerial yoga, martial arts yoga, massage and herbal supplements are excluded from coverage by many standard yoga insurance policies.

If your activities are excluded from coverage, you must contact the insurance company and purchase an endorsement".

Income Taxes

As independent contractors, yoga teachers are responsible for reporting and paying their own annual income tax. We are viewed by the IRS as self-employed and we do not have taxes deducted from our paychecks as employees do. In that light, we are also able to take business deductions from the amount we owe, which can include teacher trainings and workshops.

The subject of taxes is such a lengthy and complex issue that it deserves its own time and focus. Thus, I will not include anything more about it here. Instead, I will refer you to the eBook I've written on the topic, The Yoga Teachers' Guidebook To Income Taxes (www.loveteachingyoga.com/the-yoga-teachers-guidebook-to-income-taxes).

CHAPTER 9: CONCLUSION

"Your peers are people in the business who are going to push your forward and support you in every phase of your teaching career." – Goldie Graham

ASK FOR HELP

Don't be afraid to ask for help; you don't have to do this alone. Know that your friends and family would love to help support you. Reflect on the skills of those around you and think about who can help you and how. Ask your friend who's a graphic designer to help you with your website and marketing materials. Ask your uncle who's an accountant to help you get your bookkeeping started. Join yoga teacher groups on Facebook to ask your peers for advice and meet regularly with other teachers to just chat and bounce ideas off one another. People want to see you succeed, so they won't mind sharing their time and skills with you.

Find A Mentor

Having a mentor is one of the most important keys to success, especially early on. Mentors have insight beyond your knowledge, and sometimes there's no sense in reinventing the wheel. Just one single "ah-ha" moment with a mentor can save you months of work or prevent you from making a costly mistake. When we have awesome ideas that excite us, we often turn to our family and friends for feedback. While this can be helpful to get a "student" or "outsider" perspective, it doesn't replace advice from experienced teachers and experts in our field. Nothing beats brainstorming ideas with someone who's actually been there and done that. Not to mention, mentors usually have a more elaborate network of business connections that they may share with you when the time is right.

One of the biggest obstacles to finding and cultivating a good mentor relationship is the fear of asking busy people for their time. Expert entrepreneur, Marie Forleo, has six fabulous pieces of advice to help you overcome your fear and get the support you need.

Directly from here video on MarieTV, <u>How To Find A Mentor: 6 Steps To Get The Support You Want</u>, here's Marie's advice (www.marieforleo.com/2016/09/mentorship):

1. You do not need to meet someone to be mentored by them. You can gain from people's experience through their books, podcasts, articles, TV shows, etc.

2. Don't look for one mentor, look for many. Don't put so much pressure on one relationship, that's not wise emotionally or intellectually. If you only get advice from one person, you can miss out on learning from different points of view. No one person is going to have all the answers.

3. Don't always look up, look to the side. When you're looking for people to connect with and learn from, look to your colleagues too.

4. Be specific, not vague. When you ask questions, be as specific as you can because you're much more likely to get help on a specific problem.

5. Earn respect and trust through action. If there's someone you really want to learn from, be a true and devoted fan. Buy their books and leave reviews, take their

workshops, show up to their speaking engagements, introduce yourself and let them know how their work has impacted you. Show up in their world with a genuine, generous and non-agenda-filled heart.

6. Do great work in the world. Start building up your body of work. Be consistent. Hustle your buns off. Nobody wants to start a business relationship with someone who isn't actually doing the work. If you want someone to invest in you, give them a reason to believe in you.

HAVE COURAGE

"Courage is the commitment to begin without any guarantee of success." Johann Wolfgang von Goethe

Being courageous doesn't mean being fearless. Being courageous means choosing to act even in the presence of fear. While this book is a tremendous resource, it still comes down to you. I don't have all the answers or a magic formula. I can only guide you.

One could read every spiritual book in existence, but you know that doesn't mean one is enlightened. You have to find the courage within to put yourself out there and do the work.

At times, fear will creep in and you'll doubt yourself, but that's OK. When I first started Love Teaching Yoga, my heart was filled excitement and I was full of momentum. Yet, sometimes at night as I laid in bed, I'd begin to second guess myself. When I came upon a difficult challenge or was faced with failure, I'd feel insecure and question my abilities. Nevertheless, overcoming self-doubt is like a meditation. Just as we teach our students to gently bring their awareness back to the breath when the mind wanders, gently bring yourself back to the love and passion within. Believe in yourself and ease yourself back into that state of love and faith when fear is overwhelming you. You've got this.

Don't worry about getting it all right the first time. It's a process and your business will evolve naturally with time. Yeah, you'll fall down a few times and scrape your knees, but getting up and trying again is what separates success from failure. Falling isn't a failure, it's a learning opportunity. Giving up is failure.

I asked Anna Guest-Jelley, founder of Curvy Yoga, what's one thing she wish she knew before starting her business (www.CurvyYoga.com). This was her gracious response, "What I really wish I'd known is that building your career in any capacity is a creative endeavor. And like any creative endeavor, it requires a great level of care, detail and patience - with yourself, as well as the process. There will inevitably be things that you think will work one way that end up working another way or not at all. Also like any creative endeavor, though, that's not a sign of failure. Sometimes you just need to put a different color on the canvas, flip it upside down or get out a fresh one. This isn't a bad sign, or a sign that you're uniquely bad at what you're doing, but just part of the natural evolution of growing your own career. I now find it so freeing to remember that, and I wish I'd known it much sooner!"

People who succeed do so because they continuously put themselves out there. The more you get your hands wet, the more opportunities will come your way - things you never even imagined. Just take it one day at a time, and one step at a time. **Commit yourself to stepping forward on this path without knowing the absolute outcome.** Set a date to launch your business to the public and do your very best to be ready. Although you might not be in tip-top shape, launch what you've got and continue working on it with time. Perfection can quickly lead to procrastination and inaction. It's better to have something you can continue working on than to incessantly put it off until every little ducky is perfectly in a row. It's the little things that you do day to day that add up to success in the end, so appreciate the small wins along the way.

Even if you don't have an absolute niche carved out just yet, start with whatever is in your heart. Get as clear as you can on who you are and what you want to bring to this world, and just get started. **The only way to get better is through experience.** The confidence will come as you engage with people and begin to see the fruits of your labor. With that momentum, poise begins to outweigh fear until it no longer controls you. As Dori puts it, the courageous little fish in Finding Nemo, "Just keep swimming."

BUSINESS YIN & YANG

The universe gives you what you can handle, so when only two people show up to your first workshop, know that's exactly what you needed. In manifesting your dream career, there's a gentle blend of effort and universal faith. Yes, you most definitely have to take actionable steps that align with your goals, but you don't have to over-orchestrate the steps that get you there. There's a special place after taking action where you can then release control and let the universe do its thing. Like yin and yang, your business actions and spiritual faith may seem to be opposing forces, but are actually interconnected and complimentary. So, don't forget your yoga practice and create space for faith and love to take over. **Remember, the commitment towards your goal is what counts, so have faith and try not to overanalyze the how.**

BUILD YOUR CAREER AROUND YOUR LIFE

"Build your career around your life, not your life around your career."

Some people are happy working for security and familiarity, while others prefer creativity and independence. Neither is right or wrong, but sometimes we lose sight of our values and take on someone else's values without realizing it. Often we find ourselves joining the workforce after college and spending our lives working our way up a ladder. Between a demanding boss, emails during dinner, projects that were due yesterday, and insufficient time off, work can easily run your life instead of the other way around.

You don't have to follow or subject yourself to this path if that's just not in your heart. If you want to live with more freedom and imagination, then make it a priority to build your career around your life. When you work for yourself, doing what you love, you hold the keys to balance in your life and career. Like Courtney Mitchell from The Yoga Expo, the typical path of a yoga teacher didn't settle with her. She wanted to have a greater impact and she wanted more freedom in her life. Courtney lives by this idea of building your career around your life and is head-over-heels in love with both her life and career. You have the passion, and now your tool belt is stacked, so get out there and start creating a life and business you love. Spirit is on your side.

ADDITIONAL RESOURCES

MORE FROM LOVE TEACHING YOGA

- **Career Coaching with Michelle**
  (www.loveteachingyoga.com/career-coaching-yoga-teachers)

- **Love Teaching Yoga Podcast on iTunes**
  (https://itunes.apple.com/us/podcast/love-teaching-yoga-podcast/id1119361505?mt=2)

- **Teaching Private Yoga: Free Guide**
  (www.loveteachingyoga.com/teaching-private-yoga-2)

- **Teaching Private Yoga Starter Kit**
  (www.loveteachingyoga.com/teaching-private-yoga-starter-kit)

- **The Yoga Teachers' Guidebook To Income Taxes**

(www.loveteachingyoga.com/the-yoga-teachers-guidebook-to-income-taxes)

From Others In The Community

- **The Dailygreatness Business Planner:** an actionable journal for business planning (www.dailygreatness.co)

- **Teaching Yoga Instructional Videos** by Mark Stephens (www.markstephensyoga.com/resources/video)

- **Integrating Yoga Philosophy** with Hari Kirtana Das (www.hari-kirtana.com)

- **Delight: Eight Principles for Living with Joy and Ease** by Pleasance Silicki (www.lilomm.com/book)

- **The One Thing: A Surprisingly Simple Truth Behind Extraordinary Results** by Gary Keller and Jay Papasan (www.amazon.com)

- **Light On Law Books for Yoga Teachers & Studios** by Gary Kissiah (www.garykissiah.com)

- **How To Create and Shoot Outstanding Yoga and Fitness Content** by James Wvinner (www.amazon.com)

- **Smart Passive Income Podcast** with Pat Flynn (www.smartpassiveincome.com/podcasts)

- **Fivrr:** Find Affordable Graphic Designers, Voice Overs, Editors, Music & more (www.fivrr.com)

- **Canva:** Easily create graphic designs and documents for your marketing materials (www.canva.com)

WORKS CITED

Judie Hurtado, "Want To Be A Successful Yoga Teacher? Sadie Nardini Shares Her Secrets," Elephant Journal. August 24, 2012. http://www.elephantjournal.com/2012/08/want-to-be-a-successful-yoga-teacher-sadie-nardini-shares-her-secrets-judie-hurtado/

Dr. John F. Demartini. (2012) *Inspired Destiny: Living A Fulfilling and Purposeful Life*. Hay House, Inc.

Blueprint, "Fear Comes in Many Disguises," Printmatic Blog. January 7, 2014. http://printmatic.net/fear-comes-in-many-disguises/

http://cost-of-living.careertrends.com/l/615/The-United-States, accessed June 24, 2016.

Eric Enge, "21 Reasons You Must Become An Expert," Copyblogger. June 6, 2013. www.copyblogger.com/become-an-expert-now/

Sage Rountree, "Start Teaching Online," Yoga Journal. July 14, 2010. (www.yogajournal.com/article/teach/lights-camera-yoga).

Content Marketing Institure, "What Is Content Marketing?"
http://contentmarketinginstitute.com/what-is-content-marketing/

John Williams, "The Basics of Branding," Entreprenuer. www.entrepreneur.com/article/77408

Gary Kissiah, "Legal Essentials for Yoga Teachers and Studios," Yoga Alliance. May 20, 2014.
https://www.yogaalliance.org/Learn/Legal_Essentials_for_Yoga_Teachers_and_Studios

Made in the USA
Middletown, DE
15 December 2016